25

Diet in "Saliva" IGA
- checks
system (4x)

D0570732

Drink more H₂O

Eat Yogurt

Use Bed Blocks

Try Aloe Vera Gel - Not
Juice

Try Lactaid"

Try "Miso"

Eat Sauerkraut

Make Yogurt Pg. 121

BY THE SAME AUTHOR
The Diet-Type Weight-Loss Program

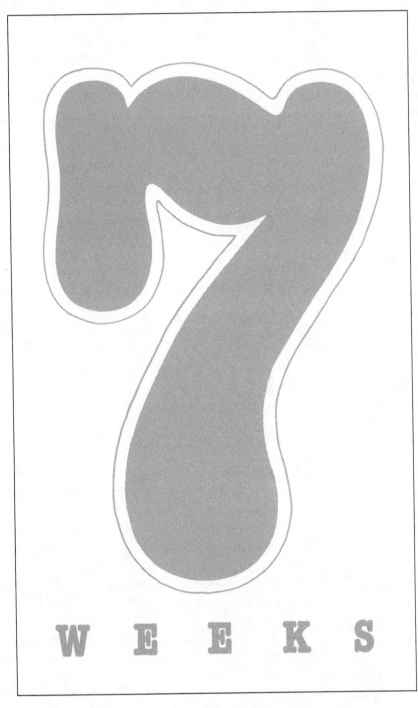

7 WEEKS

New York · London · Toronto · Sydney · Tokyo · Singapore

Seven Weeks to a Settled Stomach

*Free yourself from digestive
pain forever with the
Hoffman self-help
program*

Ronald L. Hoffman, M.D.

Simon and Schuster

Simon and Schuster
Simon & Schuster Building
Rockefeller Center
1230 Avenue of the Americas
New York, New York 10020

Copyright © 1990 by Ronald L. Hoffman, M.D.

All rights reserved
including the right of reproduction
in whole or in part in any form.

SIMON AND SCHUSTER and colophon are registered trademarks
of Simon & Schuster Inc.

Designed by Liney Li
Manufactured in the United States of America

1   3   5   7   9   10   8   6   4   2

Library of Congress Cataloging-in-Publication Data
Hoffman, Ronald L.
Seven weeks to a settled stomach: free yourself from stomach pain forever with
the Hoffman self-help program/Ronald L. Hoffman.
p.   cm.
Includes bibliographical references.
1. Indigestion—Popular works.   I. Title.   II. Title: 7 weeks to a settled
stomach.
RC827.H63   1990
616.3′32—dc20   90-33352
CIP
ISBN 0-671-68234-2

Contents

Foreword

When asked by an interviewer how he accounted for his superb health, Mohandas K. Gandhi, who subsisted on a modest vegetarian diet, is alleged to have replied that his secret was to "drink what you eat, and eat what you drink." This was taken by most observers to be a caveat to make all ingestion as slow and rhythmic as possible, but I suspect the Mahatma intended a far deeper meaning. Steeped as he was in meditative practice, he may well have been advising us to take the time at each meal to contemplate profoundly and respectfully the universal act of feeding, not merely as a ceremonial ritual of reverence and gratitude, but because, like breathing, the consumption of food and drink is such a central part of our physical survival.

Clearly, most of us do not follow the Gandhian principle (about which Dr. Hoffman has some interesting things to say in Chapter 7) because we have an attitude mingled of denial, confusion, or ignorance about the vital significance of the digestive process. Despite the burgeoning interest over the past twenty-five years in things gastronomic —from *haute cuisine* and the art of cookery to the issue of chemical fruit sprays and vegetarianism—we are still at the dawn of mass awareness and deep understanding of what we can do to promote the harmonious and enriching use of our food and drink. Moreover, we are woefully uninformed about what to do, or ask to have done to us, when the complex activities of the alimentary tract go awry. This latter point is a serious matter, since, as Dr. Hoffman rightly points out, gastrointestinal complaints are the second most frequent cause of all visits to doctors' offices. Most doctors, unfortunately, have had severely limited training in matters of nutrition; only recently have medical schools and postgraduate training programs begun to acknowledge the importance of food in the health of their patients.

Dr. Hoffman has obviously redressed that educational lapse on his own. He understands, and helps the reader to understand, exactly what goes on when we eat, what the true experts have learned about health-promoting and health-damaging foods, and most important, how we may become informed, self-reliant managers of our own digestive systems. He has made a formidable investigation of all the most talked-about issues of the day, from cholesterol and food allergies to high-fiber diet plans and mineral supplements, from synthetic antacids to colon cancer, and he guides us through this mine of information with a supportive hand. In a way that is never characterized by missionary zeal or scientific bias, Dr. Hoffman delivers a balanced and even-handed account of medical therapeutics drawn not just from Western science, but also Chinese medicine, homeopathy, yoga, self-hypnosis, biofeedback and the herbal medical tradition. And he helps us to see how foods themselves may be implicated not only in gastric distress, but in many other human discomforts and illnesses. His approach is both practical and ecumenical; he is as concerned with psychosocial and stress-related factors in digestion as he is knowledgeable about physiology and biochemistry.

Finally, and perhaps most important, Dr. Hoffman provides not only comprehensive and sensible advice but also a real step-by-step program to alleviate digestive complaints and prevent additional problems in the future. His book is a clear, succinct, and trustworthy primer on all these vital subjects.

Richard Grossman
Director
The Health in Medicine Project
Montefiore Medical Center
Bronx, New York

Your Digestive Woes

Why Your
Belly Aches

*" 'We do not live by what we eat,' says an old adage, 'but by what
we digest.' We must then digest in order to live, and this necessity
is a law which makes its power felt by rich and poor, by peasant
and king."*

—J. A. Brillat-Savarin,
The Physiology of Taste, *1825*

Most of us feel digestion's power is downright tyrannical. Quick
—guess the name of the best-selling prescription drug around the
world. No, not Valium. Not penicillin. It's Zantac, an antacid, a
drug that suppresses stomach acid. Tagamet, another antacid, used
to be the number-one drug worldwide, with annual sales up to
$1.13 billion. Now Zantac is the best-selling drug ever—$2 billion a
year!

These drugs are moneymakers because one third to one half of all
Americans suffer chronic abdominal pain. According to the National
Center for Health Statistics, at least 5 million of us have ulcers, 6
million have frequent indigestion, and another 8 million are constipated. Drug industry surveys report that 18 million of us rely heavily
on over-the-counter stomach remedies, medications that are largely
ineffective and not even entirely safe. Even so, another 50 million of

us reach for those bottles and tablets occasionally—once a week to once a month.

Digestive diseases are the third largest category of medical expenses in the United States. In 1986, Tagamet became the first drug ever to hit one billion dollars in annual sales. The market for those over-the-counter antacids, which can be worse than useless, exceeds $200 million a year. Another $50 million goes to advertise them. And the fourth most-popular over-the-counter remedy in this country is Preparation H for hemorrhoids, which usually are painful side effects of constipation.

Gastrointestinal complaints, most of them minor, are the second most frequent cause of visits to doctors' offices. Moreover, a great variety of more bothersome aches and pains elude diagnosis. At some point, after you've made the rounds of several specialists, one will tell you, "We don't know what it is. But it's not life-threatening—you're not in danger. *You'll just have to learn to live with it.*"

So most of us end up haphazardly treating our symptoms with nostrums from the corner drugstore. Some of these are ineffectual; others are downright dangerous, and none of them gets at what's really wrong. Meanwhile, we worry that our chronic digestive ailments will turn someday into something that will kill us. Occasionally we're right: chronic constipation can be a harbinger of colon cancer. Only then, when we're in really dire straits, will our digestive troubles win serious medical attention.

There are several reasons why orthodox medicine hasn't come to grips with stomachaches.

• *No one dies* of most chronic digestive disorders. Government research money for gastrointestinal problems is minimal, and there's no national center for research. Working on problems like gas or hiccups or constipation is just not considered glamorous; there are no breakthroughs.

• Thanks to the sorry state of gastrointestinal research, we don't even know exactly how the digestive system works. We're still years away from understanding the roles hormones play, for instance, or the link between your mind and your gut.

• Unfortunately, harried physicians, increasingly pressed for time to treat everyone who needs them, have succumbed to the pressure of prescribing the drugs that pharmaceutical companies pour many millions of dollars into developing and promoting. Most doctors get free samples in the mail daily; medical journals are thick with glossy ads for drugs. Doctors end up making out literally millions of prescriptions every week for drugs that don't do the stomach much good (see list of Some Scary Stats).

Prescription drugs seem like quick fixes. Sometimes they even ameliorate symptoms temporarily. But that's the rub: when prescription or over-the-counter drugs do help, they tackle symptoms, rarely the deeper roots of digestive woes.

The first step in helping any stomach problem is to change your diet. That's tough to do. Ironically, modern medicine *can* cope well with very bad cases: nowadays, high-tech procedures can forecast potentially disastrous illnesses like colon and stomach cancers. And emergency care for sudden catastrophes like bleeding ulcers and appendicitis is improving. But many digestive problems require the proverbial ounce of prevention—and in these instances, doctors are often less effective, because medical schools have not traditionally provided this kind of training.

Today, I'm happy to say that the nutritional education picture is brightening somewhat: the diet recommendations of the American Heart Association and the National Academy of Science are quite close to my own. And most medical schools are adding courses in nutrition and placing more emphasis on prevention. But too many doctors practicing today received almost no formal instruction in nutrition in medical school. I know: the only "course" I got was five lectures in the spring semester of my fourth and last year. By that point, most of us were exhausted, burned out—ready to goof off or fall in love. Almost everyone considered the nutrition lectures a gift, a—pardon the expression—"gut course" that was impossible to fail.

Once the majority of medical school graduates have started practicing medicine, they have realized the inadequacies of their education. Then they have noticed that poor eating habits underlie most patients' digestive difficulties. But by then it's too late for them to get the background they need to give adequate advice. Most new doctors don't know even the basics: what a person's nutritional needs are over a lifetime, how chronic disease affects nutrition and vice versa, or how to evaluate fad diets.

Even though most physicians may recognize that prevention is necessary, they have a very hard time going against their training. The

Modern medicine, with its emphasis on quick fixes with drugs, conspires to make your stomach ache even more often. Here's a list of drugs that can be of no help to your gut. In some cases, doctors give out over a million prescriptions *every week*. Where possible, I've listed figures for internists and obstetricians/gynecologists (OB/GYNs), because many patients use these specialists as general practitioners.

Drug	*Effect on Your Gut*
ANTIBIOTICS	Internists alone dispense 1,416,000 prescriptions every week; OB/GYNs give out another 2,645,000. Besides killing off your beneficial intestinal flora, causing digestive problems, antibiotics can impair production of vitamin K.
ANTACIDS	Internists dispense 736,000 prescriptions every week, OB/GYNs another 872,000. Besides often being ineffectual, antacids can cause constipation or diarrhea, and malabsorption of nutrients, especially iron, vitamin B_{12}, folic acid, and calcium.
LAXATIVES	OB/GYNs alone give out 760,000 prescriptions every week. Besides being habit-forming, laxatives can cause gas, diarrhea, and even rebound constipation. They can also reduce transit time and absorption of nutrients, especially minerals and vitamin D, often leading to malnutrition in the elderly.
ANTIDEPRESSANTS	Can cause nausea, constipation, diarrhea, vomiting, dry mouth, loss of appetite.

(continued from opposite page)

ANTICONVULSANTS	Can inhibit your body's ability to manufacture vitamin D, which protects you against colon cancer.
BELLADONNA AND BARBITURATES	These drugs can cause abdominal bloating.
ASPIRIN AND OTHER ANTIINFLAMMATORY DRUGS	Internists give out 1,188,000 prescriptions for antiarthritics alone every week; OB/GYNs dispense just as many, often for menstrual pain. These drugs can cause loss of appetite, vomiting, nausea, diarrhea, and loss of iron, vitamin C, and folic acid. Too much of either aspirin or other antiinflammatory drugs can cause gastrointestinal irritation and bleeding, especially if ingested with alcohol.
CHEMOTHERAPY	Can cause nausea and vomiting.
MEDICATIONS TO LOWER CHOLESTEROL	Some cause constipation, malabsorption of fat and of fat-soluble vitamins A, D, E, and K, as well as deficiency in iron, carotene, and vitamin B_{12}.
HYPERTENSION MEDICATIONS AND DIURETICS	Internists write out 2,724,000 prescriptions every week for these drugs, some of which may cause constipation or diarrhea, as well as loss of potassium, zinc, and magnesium.
ANTIDIARRHEALS	These drugs can cause abdominal bloating and even severe intestinal infection.

idea of suggesting natural therapies for digestive problems flies in the face of everything drilled into them at school. For example, antibiotics, drugs that most doctors rely on to the point of overprescribing them, are a clear cause of many gut troubles because they disrupt the delicate ecology of the intestine's natural flora. But you can hardly expect most doctors to warn you about the hazards of one of their most fundamental treatments!

Finally, because too many doctors have been conditioned to look for dramatic symptoms that they can attack with drugs or surgery, they urge patients with less-than-life-threatening problems to expect progressively worse health as their lot in life. They tell people with minor problems like gas, bloating, constipation, or chronic pain which doesn't respond to drugs that their symptoms are "natural," "psychological," or "the normal consequences of aging." *Let me say right now: you don't have to "learn to live with" chronic abdominal pain!*

The Modern Diet: Recipe for Digestive Disaster

"Tell me what you eat," wrote Brillat-Savarin, the doyen of fine dining, "and I will tell you who you are." Let's take a closer look at the true nature of America. According to a major national survey, our favorite foods include, in descending order, white bread, doughnuts, cookies, cake, hot dogs, and hamburgers. America's most popular drinks are coffee, tea, and whole milk—not even less-fatty skim milk or one-percent-fat milk. Next to the bottom of this discouraging list of our favorites I found rhubarb, a great natural remedy for constipation. In fact, in the mid-1800s, during the Opium War between the Chinese and the British, part of the Chinese strategy was to cut off the British army's rhubarb supply. Apparently the Chinese thought the British would buckle under the weight of undigested roast beef and Yorkshire pudding!

While we overlook the benefits some foods could bring us, we avidly consume fatty, sugary foods that can make us sick. In 1970, a British research team reported that Britons, subsisting on roasts and tea cakes, had a high rate of colon cancer. Meanwhile, it was rare among Africans, who ate mainly vegetables and consequently much more fiber. Up until 10,000 years ago, when we began farming, that's what most people ate.

A BRIEF HISTORY OF BRAN

👍 ————————————————————————————

• **4000 B.C.**: Prehistoric people live on low-fat, high-fiber diet of game, fish, vegetables—very few fruits and grains and no dairy products.

👍 ————————————————————————————

• **c.800–600 B.C.**: Out of respect for animals, Hindus and Buddhists embrace vegetarian diets.

👍 👎 ————————————————————————————

• **c.400 B.C.**: In ancient Greece, Hippocrates stays on the fence, intoning, "All things in nutriment are good or bad relatively." He's keen on meat, however, and recommends eggs, cheese, and particularly ass's milk.

👍 ————————————————————————————

• **c.500 B.C.–250 A.D.**: Ancient Greek philosophers Plato, Pythagoras and his disciple Porphyry favor vegetarianism. Porphyry attributes the hardiness of the warring Greek city-state of Sparta to moderate eating and drinking. He maintains that "the beginning of man's misery" was abandoning the simple life of the Pythagorean Golden Age, which featured a high-fiber diet of fruit and acorns.

👍 ————————————————————————————

• **c.30 A.D.**: Jesus may have been a vegetarian: the Essenes, a radical Jewish sect to which He may have belonged, thought Pythagoras had a point. John the Baptist, Jesus' cousin, subsisted in the desert on high-protein, low-fat locusts and honey.

(continued on page 22)

(continued from page 21)

• **c.150–200 A.D.**: In Imperial Rome, Seneca and Marcus Aurelius, obsessed with personal health and avoiding *luxuria,* endorse a high-fiber, low-fat diet of cabbage, asparagus, leeks, onions, horseradish, fish, poultry. For his part, Plutarch is against "the feeding on any flesh at all."

• **1340–1400**: In "The Miller's Tale," one of *The Canterbury Tales,* Geoffrey Chaucer invents the word "fart," a sign that gas and belching were plagues in the Middle Ages.

• **c.1494–1553**: In *Pantagruel,* François Rabelais describes just one course of a huge feast, a "gallimaufry" consisting of "different kinds of soups, salads, fricassees, stews, goat-roasts, roasts, boiled meats, carbonados, great hunks of salt beef, grand old hams . . . smoked meats, pies, tarts, a pile of Moorish couscous, cheeses, junkets, jellies, and fruit of every sort."

• **1547**: Henry VIII, king of England, dies, probably of the effects of overeating.

• **1743**: Pythagoras' dietary theories are rediscovered in Florence and London.

• **1789**: Antifiber sentiment is erroneously attributed to poor Queen Marie Antoinette of France who, historians now agree, *never* declared, "Let them eat cake."

(continued from opposite page)

• **1813**: British romantic poet Percy Bysshe Shelley decides that the Pythagorean point of view is good for health and for genius. He follows a vegetarian diet for five years, writes *A Vindication of Natural Diet*—but dies at age 30 of tuberculosis.

• **c.1824**: Sylvester Graham, American inventor of the graham cracker, advocates whole-meal breads for their "innutritous substance," his phrase for fiber.

• **1833**: In The Great Lakes region, physiologist William Beaumont writes that, based on his ground-breaking observations of the stomach in action, "Bulk is, perhaps, nearly as necessary to the articles of diet as the nutrient principle."

• **1845–1888**: Hard times for whole grains. In America, author Louisa May Alcott mocks her father's vegetarian commune in *Transcendental Wild Oats*. In London, Gilbert and Sullivan spoof "vegetable fashion" and "vegetable love" in their comic operetta *Patience*.

• **c.1884**: British writer George Bernard Shaw, arguably the wittiest bran-lover of all time, comes to the rescue, pointing out that the bull is a very strong, fierce animal, even though it eats only vegetables.

• **1890**: Dr. John Harvey Kellogg sets up a health spa in Battle Creek, Michigan, then invents bran-filled breakfast cereals like granola and shredded wheat for spa visitors.

(continued on page 24)

(continued from page 23)

- **c.1915:** Doctors denounce fiber as the cause of indigestion, cramps, ulcers, even diverticulosis; they advocate white bread.

- **1930s:** Nutritionists say there's no proof, one way or the other, that a vegetarian diet is good for you.

- **1950s:** Americans define a good meal as one that represents "the four main food groups," even though their Stone Age ancestors proved that you need only two—animal protein and wild plants.

- **1970s:** A new age dawns. British researchers, led by Dr. Denis P. Burkitt, link colon cancer to a high-fat, low-fiber diet, and coin the phrase "dietary fiber." Over the next twenty years, fiber slowly becomes fashionable again.

- **1989:** U.S. National Research Council recommends a modified Stone Age diet that is more than half vegetables, legumes, fruits, whole grains and cereals.

Consequently, some doctors and scientists have become very interested in Paleolithic people's diet. Before agriculture, our ancestors stalked wild animals and lived off the land, foraging berries, nuts, seeds, and vegetables. They traveled around in search of food, so they got a great deal of exercise and were very fit. They ate few grains and fruits, and since they had no domesticated animals, they ate no dairy products. What's more, they used no salt or alcohol, and only a very little sugar in the form of honey or tree sap. Yet our predecessors' diet was higher than ours in protein, vitamin C, fiber, and vital minerals like potassium and calcium! And judging by their self-portraits on cave walls, none of our ancestors was fat.

While agriculture and industrialization have changed our diet dramatically, our digestive system remains attuned to a caveman's diet. One investigator has dubbed us modern folk "Stone Agers in the fast lane." And because the pace of evolution is so slow, our poor digestive tract will always be sadly behind the times. No wonder it often can't work very well. Especially in the past fifty years, with the advent of processed foods and preservatives, our digestive tract has had to cope with all sorts of new, exotic chemicals and drugs—not to mention pesticides, poisons, and modern pollutants. Comedian Marshall Efron once demonstrated that "a modern lemon cream pie, factory approved," contained no lemon, eggs, or cream. It was mainly chemicals, including one used in detergent!

Perhaps you think going back to a Cro-Magnon diet to cure your stomach is pretty silly—even impossible. Maybe you're asking, "How will I get enough calcium if I avoid dairy products? And if I eat as much meat as cavemen did, won't my diet be too high in fat?"

Well, some vegetables contain more calcium than milk, and you can choose leaner poultry and game instead of well-marbled beef. In fact, you can find the equivalent of the Paleolithic diet in any well-stocked supermarket. And never fear, you will be well nourished. Early in 1989, the extremely sober, conservative National Research Council, the research arm of the National Academy of Sciences that studies technical issues for the federal government, tacitly endorsed the caveman's diet. An ideal regimen, according to the council, consists of 55 percent carbohydrates, less than 30 percent fat, and only about 15 percent protein. This is astonishingly close to a prehistoric diet, which was just a little higher in carbohydrates and protein, with 10 percent less fat. Similarly, the council's report advised laying off salt and alcohol.

Practicing Preventive Medicine

If a natural diet is better for us, why shouldn't natural remedies that also have been around for thousands of years work as well as drugs—if not better? After all, these remedies are made of herbs and plants that existed when our digestive tract was evolving, whereas drugs are a much newer feature of our biological landscape. That's a major reason why all drugs have side effects.

I first began thinking along these lines while I was still in medical school, trying to decide on a specialty. I already had gotten very interested in nutrition, and had even volunteered for a study of vegetarian students. I loved surgery, and had been told I was pretty good at it. But I worried about how I could combine it with nutrition and prevention.

Among the surgeons supervising me and other medical students was a slim, healthy-looking chief resident who regularly picked out salads in the hospital cafeteria while everyone else inhaled hot dogs, French fries, and milkshakes. I asked him why.

This surgeon told me, "In the work I do, every single day I see so many problems that are the direct result of people's not paying any attention to their diet." Here was a doctor, using stopgap surgery to stave off the consequences of his patients' decades of self-neglect. And he was urging me to concentrate on prevention. "If I could train over again," he said, "I'd focus on nutrition."

I paid attention. I went on to a residency in internal medicine, not surgery. As I began practicing, I developed my own preventive approach to digestive complaints, an approach that almost never requires intervention with drugs. Instead, I've come up with effective herbal remedies, and borrowed techniques from alternative and Eastern medical traditions. I have seen patients with gastrointestinal ailments improve thanks to acupuncture, chiropractic, massage, even yoga. Above all, I work to persuade these patients to change their diets.

Right now, most of the evidence favoring a preventive approach to digestive problems is anecdotal; a doctor notices an improvement here or reports an unusual case there. Scientists don't consider anecdotes scientific proof; clinicians also tend to distrust them. As far as most of the medical establishment is concerned, the burden is on doctors like me who favor alternative approaches to prove that they work.

However, as I'll be telling you in this book, more and more hard evidence is surfacing that demonstrates the worth of a few ounces of prevention. And I can wholeheartedly recommend these treatments because *I've tried them out myself—and they work.*

Moreover, I have watched my approach benefit thousands of my own patients. The good news about a preventive approach to gastrointestinal discomfort is you don't have to go to a doctor or a clinic to make it work; *you can do it yourself.*

It can work for you in less than two months. I'll show you my special seven-week plan that will settle your stomach for life. I'll teach you how to be a digestion detective, so you can help your own doctor help you if you need medical care for severe stomach disease.

There's no one single cure for stomach trouble. Everyone's gut needs individual care. But I'll show you how, if you follow the right food prescription for your particular condition, you can be free of chronic pain the natural way.

A Quick
Trip Down Your
Inside Tract

*"Some physiologists will have it that the stomach is a mill, others,
that it is a fermenting vat, others, again, that it is a stew-pan; but,
in my view of the matter, it is neither a mill, a fermenting vat, nor
a stew-pan; but a stomach, gentlemen, a stomach."*

—*William Hunter,*
eighteenth-century Scottish physician

D r. Hunter was insisting that the stomach, and the digestive or
gastrointestinal tract of which it's a part, is far more marvelous and
complex than any of the kitchenware that had come to other physiologists' minds. I'll never forget the first time I actually saw digestion in
progress. It was astonishing. I was a medical student watching an
operation. The patient's gastrointestinal tract was exposed, and I could
see its muscled walls moving continuously, in slow, wavelike contractions. This perpetual motion, which goes on inside you twenty-four
hours a day, is called peristalsis. It slowly propels food down your
digestive tract like ripples across water.

You can see peristalsis for yourself without going near an operating
room. Next time you spot an earthworm, look at it closely. Granted,
it's less dramatic than what I saw. Still, this segmented animal gets
around thanks to peristalsis. When it crawls, each of its segments in

turn becomes long and thin, then short and fat. In the same way, your gut moves the food you eat through your body, absorbing the nourishing parts in the process.

If you ever are lucky enough, as I was, to see digestion in action, you will be watching the old saying, "You are what you eat," come true. Your digestive tract very effectively grasps part of the outside world and turns it into your insides. Simultaneously, it protects your insides from harmful parts of your environment. If its highly efficient defenses are breached by allergy, infection, or inflammation, then your digestive tract acts like a sieve. Now, instead of being filtered out and swept from your system, allergens and toxins can pass directly into your bloodstream along with nutrients. This can happen because inflammation has enlarged the microscopic pores in your intestinal walls that normally absorb nutrients into your body.

We're all born knowing how to eat. If you tickle a newborn infant's cheek, the child's mouth will pucker in a sucking motion. Depending on where we grow up, we learn to enjoy an amazing variety of food. People can and do savor sheep's eyes, monkey brains, fish eggs, bull's testicles, insects. As is, most food is useless to the human body. What you eat has to be broken down into liquid, the nutrients extracted and then absorbed into your blood, which circulates them through your body to become its fuel. Finally, the useless parts of your food have to be eliminated.

Your digestive tract, a wonderful dis-assembly line for food, carries out this vital process. "I like to imagine," pathologist F. Gonzalez-Crussi has written, "that, aside from the prohibitions imposed by the mind, nothing in the universe—animal, vegetable, or mineral—would be rejected by man's undiscriminating stomach. Given time, we would evolve the enzymes needed to disintegrate stainless steel or to digest cast iron."

A Window on Digestion

For a long time, no one had any idea how digestion worked. People assumed that food decayed in the stomach. Then in 1822, a young Canadian trapper, Alexis St. Martin, working near the Great Lakes, was accidentally shot at close range in his left side. A U.S. Army doctor, William Beaumont, who was stationed nearby, treated St. Martin—so well that his patient lived to be 83. But Beaumont couldn't close St. Martin's wound completely. The hole provided him with a view into St. Martin's stomach, so over the next eight years, he took a series of pioneering notes on how it worked. He watched how stomach juices responded to different foods St. Martin ate, or what happened inside his belly when he was frightened or furious.

Today, many other experiments and observations later, we know more about the digestive tract's many wonderful properties. For instance, to break down food, it uses acid so powerful it corrodes metal. Your digestive tract is especially rich in lymph node tissue—part of your immune system—and it generates antibodies to defend itself. It protects you from bacteria and poisons you constantly swallow by accident. The toxins you take in —not to mention your many meals— are hard on your gut. But it heals and regenerates itself, so rapidly that you boast a completely new intestinal lining every three days. It is incredibly efficient, processing over 95 percent of what you eat. It's so efficient, in fact, that if you overeat, you gain weight! It digests protein you put into it, but even though it's made of protein, it does not digest itself. That is, unless things start to go very wrong, and then you come down with an ulcer.

Obviously, anything that interferes with this finely tuned system is going to be painful and upsetting. If you want to avoid digestive problems, I say, "Eat with your head." In ancient times, when we foraged and hunted for food, nature's supply limited the gastronomic excesses we could commit. Now that we can find dinner in a supermarket, only our reason constrains the mayhem we may wreak on our insides. In roughly the past fifty years, we have started eating new foods and chemicals—but despite fifty million years of exquisite evolution, our digestive tract is prepared for only a prehistoric diet.

Eat Smart

Actually, "Eat with your head" is superfluous advice. Eating and digestion begin in your head. They are governed by your brain and nervous system. Your brain sends signals to the many nerves lacing the well-muscled walls of your gut's sections. These signals trigger peristalsis and the other parts of the process. The mere thought of food is enough to make your mouth water—that is, to prompt the first steps of digestion: increasing the flow of saliva from the three pairs of salivary glands in your mouth, and triggering a rainfall of digestive juices in your stomach. Ivan Pavlov, the Russian physiologist, won the Nobel Prize in 1904 for discovering the brain-gut connection. Experimenting with his famous dogs, he showed how the brain and nervous system control gastric juices.

What's more, eating ends in the head, too. When you've had enough to eat, your gut sends a complex signal to your brain that gives you that sated feeling of "No more, thanks." The stomach is slow to sense that it is full; this signal takes about twenty minutes to reach the brain. One day, the natural substance that prompts the satiety signal may be sold as a safe diet pill, or perhaps electronic devices will be implanted in the satiety center, so you can feel full *before* you start a meal. Until then, eat slowly. Your digestion will work better because your stomach won't be overloaded, and you'll stay slim.

I think that if you understand how your digestion works, especially how your gut shields you from toxicity and infection, it's easier to eat so that digestion works properly. Nowadays, we still don't understand exactly how all its interesting steps work, but we do know a lot. Read on, and I'll show you how a problem with the structure or the processes of your digestive tract translates directly into a specific disorder. To paraphrase Dr. Hunter, who opened this chapter, your pain isn't a mystery; it's a stomach that can't work as well as it knows how. I've discovered that treating most stomachaches involves prevention—taking steps to *avoid* problems, to *allow* the gut to do its job right.

What Happens to a Mouthful

Look at the diagram of your digestive tract on page 33. It may look hopelessly complicated and as tangled as a plate of spaghetti. Actually, if you could unfold the 30-odd feet of your digestive tract, you'd see simply a long, straight, hollow tube with specialized sections, hooked up to some accessory organs along the way. Whenever you eat, you send your meal down this elaborate tube on a trip that averages about 36 hours—though it can take much longer. Your food—and I hope you chose a halibut over a hot dog—passes through the tube's various hollow sections, from the mouth to the esophagus, to the stomach, to the small intestine, and then to the large intestine or colon. By that time, only about 5 percent of your fish is left, to be expelled, along with living bacteria from your colon, when you defecate.

To start your halibut on its journey, you have to swallow it. Swallowing is the only part of digestion that's voluntary. The rest is automatic, controlled by your brain and other parts of your nervous system.

You swallow a piece of fish in just a few seconds, but even so, several important parts of digestion have already taken place. Your teeth have chopped your food into bits small enough to digest. Your salivary glands have exuded enough saliva to mix the morsels into a wet mush—every part of digestion is *very* wet—and your tongue and mouth have molded the food into a slick ball suitable for swallowing. Because every stage of digestion requires a good deal of water, stepping up the amount of water you drink daily is a first step to solving a digestive problem.

EXACTLY WHERE IS MY GUT?

It's higher than you think—way above your navel, in fact. Your *stomach* is under your rib cage, with its highest point very close to your heart. Your *pancreas* is also above your waist, just under and behind your stomach. So is your *liver,* to the stomach's right. The liver's lowest point is level with your bottom right rib. Even your *duodenum* is above your navel. Below it is the rest of your *small intestine.* Your *colon or large intestine* begins below your navel, on the right. Then it rises to just above your waist, crosses over to the left, and descends into your rectum.

So if you feel like you have a "stomachache," the real trouble may be in your colon. And if you complain of chest pain, something's probably gone wrong in your esophagus. Women sometimes mistake appendicitis for a gynecological problem.

If you prick your finger, you can tell exactly where the hurt is. Not so with your digestive tract. Why aren't we wired so that we're able to tell exactly where the pain is in our gut? Apparently, there was no evolutionary value in precisely locating internal distress. Evolution's approach was simple—if your insides hurt, they hurt! Exactly where was less important to your system than the warning sign of pain. I think digestive pain can be positive if it precipitates a change, such as losing weight or changing your diet, that benefits your entire digestive system.

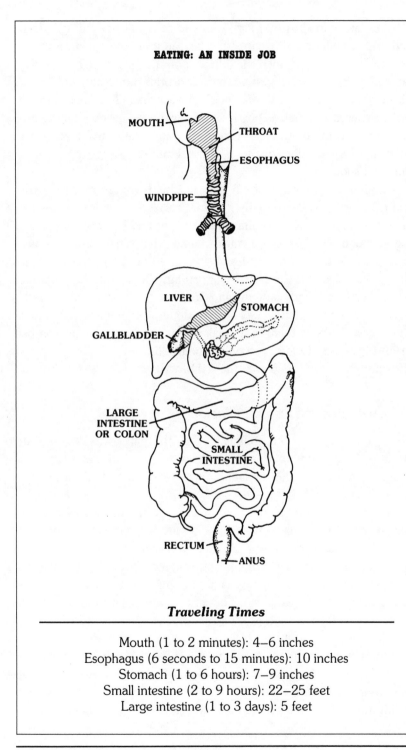

EATING: AN INSIDE JOB

MOUTH

THROAT

ESOPHAGUS

WINDPIPE

LIVER

STOMACH

GALLBLADDER

LARGE
INTESTINE
OR COLON

SMALL
INTESTINE

RECTUM

ANUS

Traveling Times

Mouth (1 to 2 minutes): 4–6 inches
Esophagus (6 seconds to 15 minutes): 10 inches
Stomach (1 to 6 hours): 7–9 inches
Small intestine (2 to 9 hours): 22–25 feet
Large intestine (1 to 3 days): 5 feet

Chew your food as thoroughly as you can. For one thing, it feels good and your food will taste better, so you'll enjoy your meal more. And studies have confirmed the folk wisdom that chewing food slowly and well means better digestion and absorption into your body. One reason is that you increase your food's surface area. That means that it can be exposed as much as possible to your gut's digestive juices, thus speeding absorption. In fact, increasing your meal's surface area is a crucial part of your digestive tract's disassembling job at every stage of your food's journey.

Another reason why careful chewing helps digestion is that you produce more saliva, especially if you're relaxed, so that your food is copiously soaked. Saliva is almost entirely water, but it does contain an enzyme, or catalyst for chemical change, that starts to break down starch into the simpler molecules of sugar. So digestion begins right in your mouth, and you can taste it happening. Chew a slice of potato or a chunk of bread long enough, and you'll notice that it turns faintly sweet. If you're ingesting any toxins along with your bread, saliva dilutes and weakens them. Saliva also contains antibodies to combat harmful invaders. In fact, certain antibodies in normal saliva are powerful enough to neutralize even the AIDS virus.

The Esophagus: Outside to Inside

When you swallow, your tongue pushes the ball of food into your pharynx. At the same time, a valve closes off your lungs and larynx— though if you try to talk or laugh and swallow simultaneously, you might cough and splutter because some food has "gone down the wrong way." Your tongue is now blocking your food's way back to your mouth so the slick ball can slide in only one direction: down into your esophagus, a muscular tube about ten inches long and one inch wide. The esophagus has a tough mucous-membrane lining, like the inside of your mouth. The esophagus's lining is your digestive tract's second defense against any toxins or harmful organisms in the descending food. Coating the food as it passes, mucus that this lining secretes also protects your esophagus from abrasive bones or seeds.

Powerful peristaltic contractions move food along the esophagus's length. Another advantage of eating slowly is that this passage, called deglutition, feels quite pleasant; it's that comfortable feeling of food settling into your stomach. Fluids and semisolid food whiz down the esophagus in about six seconds; dry food may take as long as fifteen minutes. In a healthy digestive tract, nothing fazes peristalsis, including gravity: food can reach your stomach even if you're standing on your head, or floating weightless inside a space shuttle.

The Stomach: An Acid Bath

Once peristaltic contractions have moved the food ball to the end of your esophagus, another valve opens and food squirts into your stomach. You may be surprised to learn that no absorption occurs here; the stomach is a food storage bag. Wrinkled, muscular, and pear-sized when it's empty, it grows smooth and rounded as it fills. Food stays here from three to six hours, as peristalsis kneads, churns, and mixes it with mucus and digestive juices flowing from the 35 million tiny glands in your stomach's mucous-membrane lining. These glands pour out a rain of acid—hydrochloric acid, that is—laced with another enzyme that breaks down the protein in the fish, meat, beans, eggs, or milk you've swallowed.

Your stomach is an unsung hero. It is one of the finest protective mechanisms in nature. Because most of the body is neutral or alkaline, early researchers were shocked to realize that the stomach bathes food in acid, strong enough to reduce meat to liquid and burn through skin. The stomach's acid virtually sterilizes food, killing many organisms that might infect the rest of your digestive tract. The stomach also can expel poisons in a violent muscle contraction—vomiting.

But how does the stomach protect itself? After all, it's made of protein, so why doesn't it break down its own walls? Why isn't it eaten up by its own acidic juices? Sometimes it is—that's called getting an ulcer.

Normally, the stomach has a self-protective mechanism known as cytoprotection ("*cyto-*" means "cell"). This mechanism is so strong that it's almost a force field in the "Star Wars" sense. We're not quite sure exactly how it operates, but we do know prostaglandins are at work here. These powerful chemical messengers, which blunt or trigger cellular activity, are in the thick mucous membrane that lines the stomach. They provide an active, chemical shield that buffers the stomach's walls while allowing its acid to work.

Another way prostaglandins work to protect your stomach is by constantly repairing its lining. Regular meals—never mind bacteria

---

DIGESTION MEANS CRUNCHING BIG NUMBERS

—25—

Your small intestine, a masterpiece of compact design, covers only 9 to 11 feet inside your body. But stretched out, the small intestine is up to 25 feet long. If spread flat, its lining could cover almost two tennis courts.

—40—

Your stomach can hold two and a half pints of food. You eat about two gallons every day—40 tons over a lifetime.

—50 to 250—

Your front teeth can press with as much as 50 pounds of force to break up food. Your back teeth are good for up to 250 pounds of pressure.

—70—

Your body is about 70 percent water. Blood is 90 percent water, the brain 75 percent. So is most food: bread is more than one-third water, meat over one-half.

—98—

Food can take 24 to 98 hours—and even over a week—to pass through the digestive tract. Leftovers from that big Sunday dinner may be just making their exit the following Saturday.

—100—

Over just a few hours, one salivary gland in your mouth can secrete over 100 times its own weight in water. Together, your three pairs of salivary glands produce a quart of saliva every 24 hours—so you swallow 2,400 times a day.

—9,000—

You have 9,000 taste buds, all on your tongue.

—400,000—

In the early days of gastric physiology, scientists preoccupied themselves with calculating the stomach's power to crush food. One researcher came up with 400,000 pounds per square inch.

and abrasions—continuously wear down your stomach's mucous membrane and its glandular cells—so much so that new cells start to form about eight hours after a meal.

Under normal circumstances, when food first enters your stomach, it stimulates nerve impulses that travel to your central nervous system. In turn, your system sends impulses to your gastric glands to secrete more acidic juice. That can be pretty noisy: you've heard digestive juices rumbling and gurgling inside you as your stomach contracts about three times a minute, mixing those juices with your food. Something else in your stomach makes those noises: trapped air. There's some in your stomach already, and you swallow more air along with your food, especially if you eat quickly. Some foods also contain quite a bit of air. An apple, for example, is about 20 percent air. This air can come back up as belches. And when your stomach is empty, air pressure produces "hunger pangs."

Fans of food combining, currently a popular approach to diet, insist that you should not combine certain foods at the same meal because your stomach is designed to digest only one type of food at a time. That is not so—though it is true that your stomach breaks down foods at different speeds. While protein and carbohydrates—pasta, fruit, vegetables—break down quite quickly, fats delay the time your stomach takes to empty. That's why fatty foods keep you feeling full longer. Food temperature also slows down the stomach's work. Warm food and drink take longer to leave the stomach than cold because they relax the stomach's three layers of muscles. Depression or sadness also makes your stomach sluggish.

But by the time the stomach's acid-enzyme solution and peristaltic churning have finished, your meal of halibut is unrecognizable. It has been transformed into a creamy, pea-souplike liquid called chyme. If you saw *The Exorcist,* you may have spotted chyme—the greenish liquid that spewed out of poor possessed Linda Blair. Once your fish looks like that, a ring of muscles at the stomach's lower end relaxes. One teaspoon at a time, the chyme spurts into the duodenum, the upper part of your small intestine.

The Small Intestine: Not a Bit Small and Very Powerful

The small intestine is very, very poorly named: not only is it spacious, but it subjects the chyme to its most dramatic transformations. Here is where absorption, the essential part of digestion, takes place as vital nutrients pass into the bloodstream. Here your digestive tract's accessory organs play their various parts.

Chyme enters the intestine in an acidic state, thanks to the stomach's digestive juices. But as it passes into the duodenum, it stimulates the pancreas, a small but mighty organ which secretes pancreatic juice. This juice is alkaline. It protects the small intestine by neutralizing the stomach's acids, and it creates an environment in which the pancreas's many enzymes can work well.

With astounding precision, the pancreas secretes the right enzymes in the right amounts at just the right times to break down exactly the kind of food you've eaten. Now carbohydrates and protein are ready to pass into the body. But fats need bile, manufactured by the liver, to dissolve them, as soapy water dissolves grease on dishes.

Bile, another alkaline cocktail, is formed continuously in the liver and stored in the gallbladder. Hormones—chemicals in the blood—regulate its flow to the duodenum. As chyme enters the duodenum, it stimulates the gallbladder also, which contracts, releasing bile into the small intestine. Certain parts of the bile then are reabsorbed through the small intestine's walls. Blood carries them back to the liver. The liver responds by stepping up its bile production. That process slows when the last of the chyme leaves the duodenum, as peristalsis carries it down into the intestine's lower parts.

Your feces can tell you roughly how much bile your last meal required. As bile is broken down chemically in your body, its dark yellow-green hue turns to brown, and eventually is partly responsible for the color of a bowel movement. Absence of bile results in a light, clay-colored stool. When bile ducts are blocked by an infection like hepatitis, bile passes into your bloodstream, and shows up in your complexion and the whites of your eyes, which then look yellowish.

The small intestine is lined with hundreds of velvety folds, each of which has millions of tiny, fingerlike projections called villi. This lining looks rather like fine toweling. Each villus is covered with thousands of columnar microvilli, and contains a rich supply of blood as well as a vessel of lymph, part of the lymphatic system which is responsible for absorbing fat. A single square inch of this lining has about 20,000 villi and 10 billion microvilli. The villi and microvilli increase immensely the surface of the small intestine's lining. If you could spread it flat, you'd have 540 square yards, enough for almost two tennis courts.

The small intestine has to be huge because it must absorb so many nutrients. About 95 percent of the chyme has to pass into your body. Absorption is key to good health. If you aren't absorbing nutrients properly, you aren't well. You can't compensate for malabsorption by eating more, because absorption depends on the vitality of your small intestine. If it is compromised, you may eat an enormous amount of food, yet most of it will pass right through you. On the other hand, if your small intestine is healthy and efficient, you may eat sparingly, yet you will thrive because you're absorbing as many nutrients as possible.

For food to be absorbed properly, some extremely complex chemical reactions have to take place in the small intestine. Carbohydrates and starches, whose breakdown began in your mouth with the enzyme in your saliva, become simpler sugar molecules, ready for absorption. Proteins begin disintegrating in the stomach and duodenum. In the lower small intestine, they break into their constituents: short chains of amino acids. Fats, which have been emulsified by bile in the duodenum, are now extremely tiny units called micelles. Salts and minerals, for their part, become electrolytes, electrically charged atomic particles in water that can pass through membranes. Electrolytes are critical to all of your body's vital functions.

The small intestine's muscular walls churn the chyme incessantly, while its villi sway like seaweed under water, stirring and seeking out absorbable nutrients. Some, like electrolytes, sugars, and amino acids, pass through the villi's membranes and into your bloodstream. Fats first enter the lymph vessels, which provide a conduit to the blood. From the lymph, fatty nutrients flow into your blood and enter your body's general circulation. Blood carries all nutrients, along with some digestive juices, to the liver.

Whenever you eat, your meal virtually assaults your liver, placing a tremendous load of work on it. An extremely vital organ, the liver has two very important tasks. First, it is a final conversion point for nutrients, changing them into forms your body can use as fuel. And it is a processing station with a detoxifying mechanism that will break down, separate out, and eliminate any remaining poisons. The liver is digestion's shock absorber, cleansing the blood to filter out any lingering toxic agents before they can reach the rest of your body.

All the work that the small intestine and its accessory organs—the pancreas, the gallbladder, and the liver—do on the chyme takes about three hours. By then, what's left of the chyme—only about 5 percent of what you swallowed—has reached the ileum, the end of the small intestine. At this point, the chyme's remains are indigestible, useless to the body. The small intestine has absorbed all usable foodstuffs and it is time for the chyme to move on into the large intestine and out of your body.

Each part of the digestive process starts on schedule because your digestive tract's parts communicate and relay information to each other. Your digestive tract is like a primitive but efficient animal that works inside you involuntarily, without any conscious effort on your part. We're rather like dinosaurs, who had a smaller, primitive brain in their tail: we have a second "brain" in our guts.

The Large Intestine: The Beginning of the End

Like the small intestine, the large intestine or colon is badly labeled. It is only five feet long, compared with the small intestine's roughly twenty feet. From your small intestine, chyme enters your large intestine by passing through another valve, called the ileocecal valve. Near the ileocecal valve is the appendix, a small dead end. Most physiologists say that the appendix has "no known role" in the digestive process. Surgeons may urge you to have yours removed, even if you're having an operation for another, unrelated organ like your gallbladder or uterus. They usually emphasize the trouble you may have if your appendix becomes infected or even ruptures. I prefer to believe that the appendix's role remains mysterious. We don't know its purpose— yet. Like your tonsils, it has a lot of lymphatic tissue, which normally processes allergens and infectious material.

If you could look at the large intestine's walls through a powerful electron scanning microscope, you'd see a puckered membrane with windowlike ducts, from which mucus hangs like cobwebs. Because your colon does not digest, no digestive juices flow from its membrane's ducts. But it does absorb: while mucus lubricates the passing waste, the membrane performs the colon's main chore, sopping up a great deal of water from the chyme. When you have diarrhea, it's usually a sign that something is blocking your large intestine's ability to reabsorb water.

Because your body has poured water on food during every previous stage of digestion, about two and a half gallons of water flood through your colon every day. Two thirds comes from your body itself: from saliva, gastric juices, pancreatic juice, bile, and intestinal secretions. About 80 percent of this water is soaked up in your colon. The colon takes in more water than there is blood in your body!

Although it secretes only mucus, your colon thrives with intestinal flora—bacteria, yeasts, and fungi, flourishing in a delicate ecological balance. Poised at chyme's last stop on its journey, colonic flora can find and process nutrients other parts of your digestive tract cannot. You acquired your own personal internal mulch heap soon after birth. When you're born, your digestive tract is sterile, and is gradually colonized by friendly flora you acquire from contact with your mother's skin.

From colostrum, a substance that a new mother excretes before breast milk, you also acquire antibodies, which remain in the small intestine to fight toxic invaders. If you are not breast-fed, you must make these antibodies yourself, a hit-or-miss process. Premature babies in intensive care, who are not fed colostrum and have minimal contact with their mothers, are prey to harmful strains of bacteria. So they often have diarrhea, and have to be given antibiotics, disturbing their unbalanced intestines even more.

Some useful bacteria find in the colon a warm, dark, moist home full of nutrients they can use, even if your body can't. They feed on your leftover nutrients, mostly carbohydrates, to form gas. Some of this gas is absorbed through the intestinal walls, but you do expel some along with your feces—and at some less convenient times as well! Bacteria give intestinal gas and feces their pungent odor.

But some of these bacteria actually *make* nutrients for you: for example, they synthesize vitamin K, a blood-clotting agent, from chyme. Because colonic flora is at work, your body doesn't have to expend quite as much energy. In excessive amounts, antibiotics kill off these helpful colonic bacteria, along with destructive bugs they were meant to eradicate. You should take in live cultures—by eating yogurt or supplements—to keep your intestinal flora in balance.

The Final Steps

As waste passes along your colon, losing water as it goes, it grows more and more solid. About 60 percent of its weight is still water, along with indigestibles like plant fiber, fruit skins, seeds, and old linings of your digestive tract. Here again, fiber is important to your colon. Your colon works best when it's full, and fiber keeps feces soft, helping to move them swiftly and easily. If you are an average, fiber-deprived American, your stool probably weighs between 3 and 5 ounces, while a rural African or Asian, whose diet is much higher in fiber, passes around 16 ounces of stool a day. Up to 30 percent of your stool's weight is bacterial cells, some of which would be harmful to other parts of your digestive tract.

Unless you have diarrhea, you have a bowel movement only at spaced intervals because peristalsis works differently in the colon. It doesn't go on continuously, but usually only during or soon after your meals, when fecal matter enters your colon and stimulates nerve endings in the rectal walls, starting muscle actions that result in defecation, the very last step of the digestive process. This is what a "bowel movement" means.

While you do have to be alert to where things can go wrong, I prefer to concentrate on how well the digestive tract works. If you understand and respect its delicate complexity, you can expect it to work well for you.

Don't Worry; Be Happy

An important way of avoiding digestive trouble is to pay attention to the mood you're usually in when you eat. As Dr. Beaumont noticed when he was looking into Alexis St. Martin's stomach, your head—meaning your emotions—also affects what happens in your gut. That's because your autonomic, or involuntary, nervous system has two modes, sympathetic and parasympathetic. When you're angry, tense or frightened, the sympathetic mode takes over, mobilizing your system for "flight or fight." Normally, digestion makes heavy demands on your circulatory system. But to prepare you to combat what it perceives as an emergency, your sympathetic nervous system shunts blood away from your gut to your muscles. Digestion, along with your other bodily functions, slows down, freeing your energy to ward off threats. No doubt you've noticed that when you're really frightened, or even just exercising vigorously, the last thing you want to do is eat.

But when you are relaxed and content, your system stays in the parasympathetic mode, and your gut is receptive to food. So try to eat when you're happy and calm—or at least *not* when you're also attempting to catch up on your reading or carry on a phone conversation. Some experts in Oriental medicine go so far as to say that you should be happy whenever you perform *any* natural function. I do think happiness helps at the table. If you're in a bad mood, or distracted, wait for a better moment. Concentrate on allowing the admirable digestive process to work for you, not against you.

But What If a Trip Down Your Digestive Tract Turns into a Bumpy Ride?

People with chronic digestive trouble have a tough time regarding their digestive system as *admirable*. I once saw an ad for a digestive disease foundation that showed a photograph of a young man clutching his stomach. Its caption read, *"I hate my guts!"* If you have chronic pain in any part of your digestive tract, that's probably just how you often feel.

Let's look at what can go wrong where, and why. If, for example, you feel pains in your chest that signal heartburn, the real problem is in your esophagus. Peristalsis, the mechanism that normally moves food in one direction only—down your esophagus and into your stomach—is failing, and food is forcing itself back up your esophagus. That's why the old-fashioned, low-tech remedy of bed blocks, so that you can sleep with your head higher than your feet, can help heartburn sufferers.

Heartburn is all too common. More than 61 million Americans suffer from heartburn monthly, and attempt to relieve it by spending hundreds of millions of dollars on antacids. The real cause of heartburn is usually obesity, stress, or the wrong diet. In short, a key part of the digestive system breaks down because of our modern way of life. The esophagus is just not designed for what we're doing with it.

Another site of frequent digestive trouble is your stomach. As I mentioned, your stomach is constantly processing your meals. So its lining needs continual repair, a job normally handled very efficiently by prostaglandins. If your stomach begins to secrete too much acid, the stomach's lining wears down, and you feel the pangs of indigestion. Or if the acid eats right through the lining's mucous membrane, you have an ulcer—literally a hole in your stomach. Some drugs, notably aspirin and other arthritis remedies, can wear holes in your stomach because they stop your body from producing prostaglandins, thus interfering with cytoprotection.

Similarly, disturbances in the delicate and exact functioning of your digestive tract's auxiliary organs are closely linked to gallbladder disease, prevalent in Western countries with rich diets. And crash dieters tend to have gallstones because the change in their eating habits alters their liver's metabolism. It has been revved up to produce a great deal of bile that usually passes out of the body. But when you suddenly start eating less, bile accumulates and may solidify into gallstones.

While one auxiliary digestive organ, the liver, already has enormous responsibilities, we tend to burden it even more. When we compound the assault an ordinary meal makes on our liver by eating junk food or taking drugs, we strain this overworked organ's capacity. If you're overweight because you overeat, and you have elevated cholesterol levels, you also may have mild liver abnormalities. Because your liver has to cope with large amounts of excess nutrients and toxic by-products, it's showing signs of overwork. When you adopt a more reasonable diet, your liver abnormalities disappear.

Every digestive disorder and disease interferes with the principal job of the small intestine—absorbing nutrients into your body—and leads to malabsorption. But sometimes medications and surgery do, too. For example, the intestinal bypass, now a discredited form of surgery for obesity, interfered with absorption so much that its recipients came down with chronic diarrhea, kidney stones, and even reduced night vision because they were not absorbing enough vitamin A.

While the small intestine is porous to nutrients, it must block toxins from entering your bloodstream. Your small intestine's mucous-membrane walls have specific places called Peyer's patches that produce antibodies to ward off foreign invaders. These intruders, such as parasites or bacteria that cause "Montezuma's revenge," or traveler's diarrhea, are capable of injuring the small intestine's lining, as they do the stomach's, so that you suffer indigestion. An inexpensive "spit test," or saliva analysis, which measures salivary immunoglobulin A, a defensive antibody that lines all your body's mucous membranes, is a good way to check on the condition of your small intestine's immune system.

From your small intestine, your food passes through the ileocecal valve into your large intestine, the last leg of its thirty-foot journey down your gastrointestinal tract. If you suffer from irritable bowel syndrome, a chronic digestive disorder accompanied by painful spasms, diarrhea or constipation, chances are your ileocecal valve functions spasmodically, perhaps because you're under stress or eating the wrong diet.

Near the ileocecal valve is your appendix. If you've ever had any sort of operation in that general area, you may have heard your surgeon suggest, "Let's have your appendix out. It's not troubling you now, but it may later." However, unless your appendix is already inflamed, removing it may be a *very* bad idea. It is made of lymphatic tissue, and some researchers note a higher rate of lymphatic cancer in people who have had appendectomies. Dr. George Crile, former chief of surgery at the prestigious Cleveland Clinic, has successfully treated cases of appendicitis, even some patients whose appendix had ruptured, with antibiotics only. After that, he became "convinced that appendectomy was not a necessary or even an effective treatment for appendicitis" if antibiotics were available.

I tend to think that serious digestive emergencies like appendicitis or gallbladder infections arise because we have interfered with the way each part of our gut "talks" to the others. One way we interfere is by trying to control digestion's involuntary processes. Sometimes our modern patterns of eating and defecating at "regular" times are at odds with the workings of our gut, and mess them up. Or we feed into the digestive tract much too much medication meant to deacidify or tranquilize it.

Eventually, after enough interference, the gut stops "talking"— and you come down with a serious digestive illness. Then you have an operation to "improve" your digestive tract or to eliminate parts a doctor may think are useless or outmoded. I'm continually amazed by how few people still have an intact gut. Frequently your operation turns out to be another intrusion that discombobulates your digestion even more.

If an operation or illness requires you to take antibiotics, your medicine will kill off destructive bugs—but also the friendly bacteria that thrive in your large intestine, or colon, making key nutrients for you. You need to ingest live cultures, by eating yogurt or supplements, to keep your intestinal flora in balance.

Like all living things, the cells that make up your large intestine's walls have to eat to stay well. Some new research has found that intestinal cells thrive on calcium and also eat short-chain fatty acids. Normally, you ingest calcium in your food, but not short-chain fatty acids. Rather, they result when bacteria break down fiber in your colon. If your colonic bacteria—and consequently their by-products, fatty acids —are depleted, your colonic mucosa (mucous membrane) becomes inflamed. If it remains chronically inflamed, you may suffer from ulcerative colitis, a serious illness. Worse yet, some new research suggests, you may be prone to colon cancer. Clearly, eating lots of calcium and fiber will help keep you and your colon in good shape.

As your small intestine does, your large intestine has to shield your body from harmful organisms in your food. As mentioned previously, up to 30 percent of your stool's weight is bacterial cells, some of which would be harmful elsewhere, including the other end of your digestive tract. If you have diarrhea, especially traveler's diarrhea, alien bacteria probably have invaded your intestines. There the toxins they release may stimulate more powerful peristalsis than usual, a natural method of ridding your body of these poisons and the invading bacteria as well.

Diarrhea, then, is not a disease, but a sign that the digestive tract is defending itself by coating invaders with mucus and antibodies, and then flushing them out. Because this self-defense preempts absorption, your feces are watery, and you feel debilitated and very thirsty. You should drink a lot to replace the water you've lost. Infants need chicken soup, thin vegetable broth, or Pedialyte, a solution that replaces crucial minerals.

Like diarrhea, constipation is a symptom, not a disease. Too little fiber in your diet can lead to constipation. If you ignore peristaltic contraction and try to hold back feces, you'll also become constipated. The longer stools stay in the colon, the drier they become and the harder to pass. The pressure of retained stools can pocket the colon's wall with small ruptures, a condition called diverticulosis. If any rupture becomes infected, you have diverticulitis, and probably are in a great deal of pain.

Sometimes you may have the impression that a meal "went right through me," but this is rare in adults. At the very fastest, a meal's transit through your digestive tract takes 24 to 36 hours. If you've ever fed a baby, however, you know that very shortly thereafter, you'll have to change a diaper. Babies do have a gut response called the gastrocolic reflex. When infants eat, a very rapid signal short-cuts through the rest of the gut and prompts defecation. As you grow up, you learn to suppress this signal through conscious control. But sometimes this powerful primitive reflex does reassert itself in adulthood, in symptoms of irritable bowel syndrome.

Listening to Your Gut

I wrote my first book, *The Diet-Type Weight-Loss Program,* because so many patients said to me, "Doctor, give me a specific diet. Tell me what to eat, and what not to eat." If I simply said, "Well, eat until you feel full," patients would say, "How much is that? Exactly how much should I eat?"

Many of us are so out of touch with our digestion that we've lost the ability to detect its signals. We can't even tell when we're satisfied! No wonder we pay little attention when our gut tries to tell us that we're mistreating it. In this book, I will show you how to translate what your gut is saying. Learn to listen to your gut. It knows what it needs.

Starting in the next chapter, you will learn to hear your gut talking as you follow the Hoffman Program, which will settle your stomach within seven weeks. As I'll be telling you on the next page, the first step is incredibly easy: you just do . . . less.

The Hoffman Program:

*Seven Weeks
to a
Settled Stomach*

The program I'm about to outline is very simple. You don't need any extra money or any special equipment—just a little time and care. Basically, you're setting out to learn how what you eat affects the way you feel.

If your gut bothers you at all—maybe you have indigestion, bloating, cramping—your first step is to start keeping a food diary. At the end of each day, jot down in a notebook what you ate at each meal and snack, and how you felt at the time, physically and emotionally. If you aren't sure what I mean by this, slow down and start paying attention. Maybe you're gulping down what you eat so quickly, or you're so distracted during meals, that you've stopped noticing how food affects you.

Don't leave anything out of your diary. Don't bother recording amounts, but do be honest. You don't have to show this to anyone, although if you have a chronic problem, you may want to go over your records with your doctor eventually. Right now, you're just tracking your daily diet's makeup and how it makes you feel.

This diary will help you with step one of the Hoffman Program: finding out *what not to eat*. When you put your meals on paper, your dietary sins, the food and habits you need to ease up on or eliminate altogether, are easy to spot.

In short order, your food diary will show you your patterns. Do you grab some junk food when you're in a hurry? Do you succumb to fatty foods, especially at parties, when you can't pass up hors d'oeuvre trays of cheese and smoked salmon? How often do you pick fresh fruit for dessert? Your diary will help you figure out whether you're committing one of the Seven Deadly Diet Sins: eating too much sugar or artificial sweeteners, coffee, fat, alcohol, or junk food. If you do any of these things, or you smoke, you probably have periodic abdominal pain. Chances are, then, that you're also guilty of the Seventh Sin, reaching for antacids. Yes, your medicine really is no good for your gut. In the long run, it can be downright harmful.

Weeks One and Two: Cut Down or Cut Out

"Many are the causes of ill health, but the principal one is the variety and excess of food."

—*from* An Easy Way to Prolong Life by a
Little Attention to What We Eat and Drink,
by a Medical Gentleman, 1775

To settle your stomach for good, first you have to erase any dietary bad habits your diary has helped you spot. This part of the Hoffman Program takes two weeks. You'll need Week One to cut down or cut out food offenders, and Week Two to start feeling better.

The First Deadly Diet Sin: Smoking. Cut It Out.

Thanks to former Surgeon General Everett Koop's campaign, you probably know very well that smokers can succumb to several deadly diseases, including lung cancer, emphysema, and heart disease. As many as one third of all cancers can be traced to smoking. Some of these cancers involve the gastrointestinal tract. The scariest statistic associated with smoking is its clear link to pancreatic cancer. A swift and painful killer, it is also one of the forms of cancer against which medicine has made the least progress.

But you may not realize that smoking affects digestion in other ways:

• Smoking appears to alter your liver's ability to process drugs, alcohol, and other toxins. You may need more medication to treat an illness. If you smoke *and* drink too much, smoking can aggravate liver disease.

• The more you smoke, the higher your chances of developing an ulcer, especially a duodenal ulcer. An ulcer means that gastric acids are eating through the mucous membrane lining your gastrointestinal tract. Because your lining can't regenerate itself quickly enough, your digestive tract starts devouring itself. If you develop an ulcer and keep on smoking, your ulcer will heal more slowly.

• Smoking contributes to heartburn, a particularly common gastrointestinal complaint.

• Smoking seems to interfere with your body's ability to absorb nutrients and use food efficiently. Some studies have found that smokers actually eat *more* than nonsmokers—despite cigarettes' reputed ability to curb your appetite. But they weigh *less* because nicotine accelerates their metabolism, interfering with absorption of nutrients.

• Chewing tobacco is just as dangerous: you risk developing cancer because you absorb large quantities of nicotine through your saliva and mouth tissues.

ULCERS

When stomach acid acts on a weakened mucosa, ulcers are the result. Normally, most of this acid is buffered by food you eat. Some researchers have found that smoking reduces the amount of bicarbonate your pancreas produces, interfering with the way acid is usually neutralized in your duodenum.

There's also some evidence that steady smoking may increase the amount of acid your stomach secretes, and speed up the rate at which it empties its acid-filled contents into your small intestine. That would explain the high number and slower healing of ulcers in smokers, as well as their inability to process food efficiently.

ESOPHAGEAL TROUBLE

When your lower esophageal sphincter, the valve that separates the esophagus from the stomach, is weak, it may allow gastric juice to reflux, or flow backward, into your esophagus. If your esophagus's lining comes into contact with too much gastric juice for too long, you feel burning pain in your chest. That's heartburn.

Certainly heartburn strikes nonsmokers occasionally. But smoking may weaken your lower esophageal sphincter and also directly damage your esophagus, so that you are more susceptible to reflux. And smoking also seems to promote the movement of bile from your intestine to your stomach. It makes reflux more harmful, because too much bile may be carcinogenic.

According to one theory, bile acids can be dangerous because they remove the surface layer of cells in your gastric lining. These have to be replaced with new cells, which grow more rapidly. These growing cells are vulnerable to cancer-causing chemicals—in food or in cigarette smoke. In this way, smoking creates a vicious circle that can lead you to esophageal or stomach tumors, especially if you mix smoking and alcohol.

WHAT IF YOU STOP SMOKING?

Some of smoking's effects on your digestive tract do seem to be short-lived. Within a half hour after you stop smoking, your pancreas's production of bicarbonate becomes normal, and your liver also functions properly again. Scientists suspect that most other digestive abnormalities are also erased soon after you stop smoking.

So, you should add your digestive health to the long list of arguments you've already heard against smoking. If you're a heavy smoker, I realize that quitting is no easy task. According to former Surgeon General Koop, smoking is as powerful an addiction as heroin. Try a group program like Smoke Enders, where you'll have the benefit of other people's support and a technique that allows you to withdraw from tobacco gradually.

Even slow withdrawal can be very unpleasant. One way to ease the pain is with Nicorette, nicotine chewing gum. Be warned, though, that it can upset your stomach. Another alternative is an ingenious use of clonidine patches, normally a remedy for high blood pressure. Many smokers struggling to quit complain of a rushing feeling that makes them long for a cigarette to clear their head. Clonidine patches may relieve that feeling—although one recent study disputes their effectiveness—without causing indigestion in the process. Apply a silver-dollar-sized patch to your shoulder or stomach for about a week.

You also will have an easier time giving up smoking if you stop drinking coffee as well. A new study has found that there's a reason why smokers sit and drink cup after cup of coffee. While smokers tend to drink more coffee than nonsmokers, they clear it from their systems faster. Caffeine remains in the blood of smokers for two to three hours, half the time it is found in the blood of nonsmokers. So if you quit smoking, but keep drinking the same amount of coffee, concentrations of caffeine in your blood will rise sharply and exacerbate symptoms of tobacco withdrawal like nervousness and insomnia.

And if you are worried about gaining weight once you quit smoking, here is some consolation from new research. According to a recent study, weight gain above the hips—a potbelly, in other words—indicates poor health and poor cardiovascular conditioning. There are different kinds of fat cells, and those that tend to accumulate around the waist are associated more with metabolic imbalances that can lead to heart disease. On the other hand, extra pounds below the hips—the pear shape associated more with a female pattern of weight gain—are less of a threat to health. This type of fat cell is associated with a lower incidence of hypertension, diabetes, and abnormal cholesterol levels—and hence a lower risk of a heart attack. In short, what counts is not how much extra poundage you have, but where it is. Smokers do tend to weigh less, but the weight you kept off while you were smoking was largely below your waist. The alteration in your waist-to-hip poundage left you more vulnerable to illness. Now you're absorbing nutrients your system has been lacking all along.

Still, I do understand that if you've stopped smoking and gained weight, the idea that you probably needed a few more pounds is no consolation. But now you may have more strength for exercise, which should stabilize your weight. Working out regularly and eating sensibly ought to prevent you from putting on too many pounds.

The Second Sin: Coffee. Cut It Down.

As you can see in the accompanying list (America's Eating Habits), coffee and tea top the list of beverages Americans drink most fre-

AMERICA'S EATING HABITS:
EXPRESSWAY TO A STOMACHACHE

In 1985, a nationwide survey found that Americans prefer their saturated fat in the form of hamburgers, and their cholesterol in eggs and steaks. In descending order, here are the 15 foods Americans love most, and the abdominal trouble they can start.

Favorite Food	*Problem It Can Give You*
COFFEE AND TEA	Rob you of cytoprotection and nutrients; speed up peristalsis, which may bring on diarrhea.
WHITE BREAD, ROLLS, CRACKERS	No fiber; lots of fat.
MARGARINE	Terrible for your arteries! and contains dangerous hydrogenated fats.
WHOLE MILK	Too much fat.
DOUGHNUTS, COOKIES, CAKE	Sugar plus fat = weight gain, increased risk of gallbladder disease.
SUGAR	Helps yeasts take over.
GREEN SALAD	Great if the dressing is sugar-free—unless you have diarrhea, when salads can be the worst!
REGULAR SOFT DRINKS	Lots of caffeine and sugar.
CHEESES, EXCLUDING COTTAGE CHEESE	Low-fat cheese is rare.

(continued on page 56)

(continued from page 55)

EGGS	If you have cardiovascular trouble, more than one or two a week is too much cholesterol.
MAYONNAISE, SALAD DRESSINGS	Hidden sugar.
HOT DOGS, HAM, LUNCH MEATS	Too much fat.
ALCOHOLIC BEVERAGES	Strip your gut lining.
HAMBURGERS, CHEESEBURGERS, MEAT LOAF	Beef is very fatty.
POTATOES, EXCLUDING FRIED	Fine without butter and sour cream.

Farther down this list of favorites are French fries, salty snacks, nondairy creamers, cold cereals, and diet soft drinks.

quently. Both coffee and tea contain a drug, caffeine. Their popularity makes caffeine the most widely consumed drug in the country.

Our primary source of caffeine is coffee, although caffeine also crops up in some surprising places (see later listing Hidden Caffeine). So far, studies have failed to link coffee to cancer, especially of the bladder or pancreas, or to heart disease. One study has found a connection between coffee and spontaneous abortion, or miscarriage, and so pregnant women might do well to reduce caffeine consumption, at least temporarily.

Once we thought coffee was good for digestion. Here's the opinion of *The New Family Receipt Book* of 1824:

"Coffee accelerates digestion, corrects crudities, removes colic and flatulence. It mitigates headaches, cherishes the animal spirits, takes away listlessness and languor and is serviceable in all obstructions arising from languid circulation. It is a wonderful restorative to emaciated constitutions and highly refreshing to the studious and seden-tary."

Today we're a little less sanguine about coffee. We know now that the oils that contribute to the distinctive flavors of coffee and decaffein-ated coffee can affect digestion powerfully—more powerfully than caf-feine does in other forms.

- In reasonable amounts, coffee enhances peristalsis, which can be helpful. Many people "can't get going" in the morning without coffee: they can't have a bowel movement until they've had their morning cup. Coffee also stimulates water secretion from the small intestine, which has a laxative effect. Some colonic-health enthusiasts rely on coffee enemas to flush out excess bile and gallbladder secretions and to detoxify the liver. All this is fine—in moderation. Peristalsis has its own pace. If you drink too much coffee, you'll get intestinal spasms.
- Whenever caffeine enters your stomach, it stimulates the flow of gastric juices. But the flavor oils in coffee and decaf are stronger stim-ulants of acid secretion than caffeine. Acid output resulting from coffee is particularly acute if you're already under stress—which means that your stomach is already pumping extra acid. This surplus acid can make ulcer symptoms worse, but there's no evidence that coffee causes ulcers in people. But like some other drugs, coffee blocks prostaglan-din production, weakening cytoprotection and perhaps leading to ul-cers.
- Coffee does seem to have a bad effect on nutrient absorption. Coffee drinkers lose vital minerals, including magnesium and calcium. Especially if you're older, this malabsorption can mean weaker bones and, in women, osteoporosis.
- Too much coffee, even decaf, raises cholesterol levels, which tea and caffeinated colas don't seem to do. Brewed coffee and decaf seems to do more damage than drip.
- Like chocolate, which also contains caffeine, coffee may exacer-bate heartburn.

SLOWING TO A HALT

Because everyone reacts to caffeine differently, no one has been able to set an "absolutely safe" limit. If you like coffee, the best thing to do is to limit your intake to that morning cup. If you're drinking several cups right now, cut down slowly. By going cold turkey, you'll suffer severe headaches and other withdrawal symptoms.

HIDDEN CAFFEINE

Beverages	Caffeine (milligrams)
Brewed coffee (6 oz.)	60–150
Espresso (3 oz.)	60–150
Cappuccino (6 oz.)	60–150
Instant coffee (6 oz.)	40–100
Tea (6 oz.)	40
Cocoa (6 oz.)	9
Cola (12 oz.)	42
Dr. Pepper (12 oz.)	41
Mello-Yello (12 oz.)	52
Mountain Dew (12 oz.)	54

Sweets	
Milk chocolate (1.65 oz. bar)	10
Chocolate syrup (2 tbsp.)	5

Pain Relievers	
Excedrin	65
Anacin	32
Vanquish	33

Watch out for Jolt, a new soft drink that contains more sugar and caffeine than Coca-Cola!

First, try avoiding all sources of extra caffeine (see accompanying list). And then try passing up one cup of coffee a week until you reach your goal of one cup per day. If you still have indigestion or cramps, you may have to give up coffee entirely. Tea may allow you caffeine's lift without coffee's side effects. But if you're prone to irritable bowel syndrome, tea may affect you adversely, too. Try not to reach for a headache remedy that contains caffeine. Yes, your headache will vanish, but your withdrawal will be set back.

Just like tobacco or alcohol, caffeine is a powerful drug. Don't berate yourself if you find giving it up a struggle. Some people mistakenly fall back on sugar to wake themselves up, but new research at the Massachusetts Institute of Technology has found that the popular notion of sugar as "quick energy" is a misconception. Sugar may seem to perk you up briefly, but this effect seldom lasts for very long. Because sugar prompts the release of serotonin, a sedating chemical, from your brain, it actually makes you relaxed and drowsy. A strenuous exercise class is a better, less-fattening alternative.

The Third Sin: Alcohol. Cut It Down.

Alcoholic beverages are America's fifth favorite choice of drink, after coffee and tea, milk, and nondiet sodas. You may wonder what's wrong with that, considering some scientific evidence that a daily cocktail or glass of wine or beer helps you relax and, in the long run, fend off heart disease.

You may think that because alcohol is legal if you're an adult, it's quite safe. But alcohol is a drug, whose effects on your body can be great. It acts on every cell because it is found wherever there's water inside you—in other words, throughout your body.

TOO MUCH IS TOO MUCH

First consider whether you drink to excess. Alcohol abuse has reached epidemic proportions in this country. About 18 million Americans have drinking problems; only about 1 million seek treatment. Even if you are not a problem drinker, I'd say that if you drink every day, you're drinking too much.

Alcohol's effect on public health is enormous: it is *the* major cause of malnutrition in otherwise healthy people. It induces loss of appetite, which leads to vitamin and mineral deficiencies and subsequently to stomach and intestinal inflammation, liver disorders, and inability to digest dairy products.

Not long ago, a patient asked me whether he should give up drinking three beers a day. After all, he ate only health food. Here's what I told him: Even if you eat well, heavy drinking may cause malnutrition because it can damage the intestinal lining, reducing absorption of nutrients. This damage can eventually lead to ulcers or worsen any abdominal trouble you already have. And since alcohol can injure your pancreas, it may interfere with your body's ability to use some vitamins and minerals.

Alcohol is tolerated by people's guts differently, but in over 40 percent it is quite irritating. Basically, it strips your intestinal lining. If you combine drink with aspirin or nonsteroid antiinflammatory or menstrual drugs like Advil or Naprosyn, or if you take Alka-Seltzer, which contains aspirin, for your hangover, you are adding more injury. These drugs erode cytoprotection, so you'll get gastritis along with your hangover.

If you drink too much, you may be more sensitive to some foods because your damaged intestinal wall no longer blocks allergens from finding their way into your system. Alcohol also poisons the friendly flora in your colon. Like weeds, other organisms overrun your internal garden, giving you gas, diarrhea, and frequently yeast infections (for more about these, see the next section on sugar).

As a result, unfortunately, some Alcoholics Anonymous meetings may be hazardous to your gastric health. Although they are the only way most problem drinkers can kick their habit, the well-sugared coffee and doughnuts often featured at these gatherings only fertilize the weeds that alcohol has fostered in your colon. Some of my patients report that more AA meetings are now conscious of the importance of diet. To discourage unfriendly organisms, you need a low-sugar diet, as well as a visit to your doctor for an antifungal treatment like nystatin. If you go to more traditional AA meetings, take carrot sticks to munch on, along with a bottle of mineral water.

"BUT I ONLY DRINK ONCE IN A WHILE!"
Use your food diary to trace the consequences for your digestive tract. An occasional glass of wine can be good for digestion: wine stimulates saliva and hydrochloric acid production, and relaxes you so that you eat more slowly. But do you have a headache or an upset stomach or diarrhea the day after only one or two drinks?

• *Indigestion:* If liquor stimulates the release of too much gastric acid, you will have an upset stomach. And because alcohol is an irritant, it can foster ulcers and exacerbate any chronic abdominal problem you may have.

• *Diarrhea:* Prolonged drinking can give you diarrhea in two ways. First, too much alcohol decreases production of pancreatic enzymes that break down food. Many alcoholics even come down with pancreatitis. Then, because fat is not being completely absorbed, the excess acts like good old-fashioned mineral oil—your grandmother's remedy for constipation. It cleans you out, and you have an attack of diarrhea.

Finally, since too much alcohol may damage your colon's lining, it can lose its ability to reabsorb water in your food. Your large intestine fills with water, giving you diarrhea.

If you're watching your weight, alcohol is a hazard: not only is it highly caloric, but for some people it tends to stimulate overeating. I'm not opposed to an occasional toast, but in general, alcohol isn't worth the trouble it can give you and your stomach.

If you decide to stop drinking, you may find that your friends and family don't take your decision very seriously. They may try to talk you out of it or ply you with drinks at every opportunity. You can always say you've discovered you're allergic. Or you can joke that half the world—the Moslem, Buddhist, and Hindu half, that is—doesn't drink. A recent poll found that in France, a country synonymous with fine wine, only 28 percent of citizens take wine regularly with meals, and another 28 percent never touch a glassful.

Finally, you're welcome to blame me: just say you're having stomach trouble and your doctor has advised you to lay off for a while.

The Fourth Sin: Sugar. Cut It Down.

In December 1988, an exhibition at the American Craft Museum in New York City featured all the intricate, beautiful ways we use sugar to celebrate life's important events. There were holiday goodies from all over the world, along with wedding cakes, sugar-coated almonds to celebrate a baby's birth, a one-and-a-half-foot-high lollipop, a fifteen-foot arch of candy rainbow, a portrait of Miss Liberty in jelly beans. Sugar on important days is one thing *but*—and I hate to sound like a wet blanket—we've become so hooked on sugar that we can barely get away from it.

In *Sugar Blues,* William Dufty's hard-hitting history of our national addiction to sugar, the author described his first attempt to get clean:

"I threw all the sugar out of my kitchen. Then I threw out everything that had sugar in it, cereals and canned fruit, soups and bread.

Since I had never really read any labels carefully, I was shocked to find the shelves were soon empty; so was the refrigerator."

Dufty had stumbled onto the truth about most modern packaged foods. They contain sugar in one of its many forms: sucrose (table sugar), fructose (in fruits, vegetables, and high-fructose corn syrup), glucose or dextrose (in honey, vegetables, and high-fructose corn syrup), and lactose (in milk).

HIDDEN SUGAR

Sugar also shows up constantly as a sweetener and preservative in packaged food. Some cold cereals are as much as 65 percent sugar. The comedian Marshall Efron once described Froot Loops as "so sweet it could be called the first breakfast dessert." Even seasonings like mustard, mayonnaise, ketchup, and commercial salad dressings contain sugar. Whether the label says maple syrup, maltose, molasses, sorghum, sorbitol, or—in health foods—more "natural"-sounding black-strap molasses, brown sugar, raw sugar, barley malt, or turbinado sugar, it's *all* sugar. The Food and Drug Administration (FDA) estimates that each of us consumes about 80 pounds of sugar every year. (I wonder who's eating the 79.5 pounds I *don't* eat.) And, of course, some of us consume far more than the national sugar average: typical American teenagers, for example, consume nearly twice their own weight in sugar annually!

WHAT'S WRONG WITH SUGAR?

The Sugar Association (sugar growers' trade association) recently began a $3 million a year television ad campaign, aimed especially at mothers, praising the "sweet, pure, and natural" benefits of homemade sugary desserts. But sugar has no nutritional benefits—no significant amounts of fiber, vitamins, or minerals. Whether it comes from cane or beets or corn or beehives or maple trees, sugar contains only "empty calories"—no nutrients. In your body, it converts into glucose, which circulates in your bloodstream, carrying calories to cells.

My main objection to sugar is that it turns your gastrointestinal tract into a fermenting vat. It's quite easy to see for yourself what I'm talking about. Take a mouthful of food that's high in carbohydrates—rice or pasta, perhaps—and chew it up thoroughly without swallowing, so that the food mixes with your saliva and some digestive enzymes. Put this wad of chewed-up food in a jar, sprinkle some sugar on it, and leave the sealed jar in a warm place overnight.

The next morning, open the jar. As you unscrew its lid, you'll hear a pop!—because you're releasing gas. Because of the sugar, your food has fermented, forming gas. This is the process you fuel in your stomach when you consume sugar. Small wonder that when you have painful gas, bloating, and even ulcers, sugar is often the culprit.

SUBSTITUTES FOR SUGAR

If you turn to artificial sweeteners, you do so with FDA approval, but at your own risk. Saccharin studies have linked the substance to bladder cancer. So far, though, public outcry has thwarted FDA attempts to ban it. Aspartame, sold as NutraSweet, is dangerous for the rare person who cannot metabolize it properly.

More important, NutraSweet, along with other nonnutritive sweeteners, doesn't do its job: it can actually increase your appetite, so that you put on weight. Taking too much of another popular sweetener, sorbitol, can give you nagging, wasting diarrhea. The FDA has approved a new sweetener, acesulfame-K, marketed as Sunette. But during testing, it produced a higher-than-usual number of tumors in lab animals, as well as elevated cholesterol levels.

"NATURAL" SUGAR

Sometimes patients protest, "I'm *not* eating sugar. I eat fruit and drink fruit juice. That's healthy, right?" No, not in excess: fructose comes from fruit, but it's still sugar. You may gain weight and, besides, a great many people have difficulty digesting sugar, even lactose and fructose. If you're susceptible to fructose, you may suffer diarrhea and stomach upset, the same kind of reaction you may have to milk if you cannot tolerate lactose. You'll learn more about food intolerances like these during the next two weeks of the Hoffman Program.

Food and beverage companies are adding more and more fructose to your diet every year in the form of high-fructose corn syrup, a combination of fructose and glucose. In 1975, the average American consumed about five pounds of high-fructose corn syrup; ten years later, that figure had jumped to forty-five. Today, the total is probably even higher, thanks to high concentrations in soft drinks.

There are some intriguing theories about the long-term health effects of boosting your fructose intake. Dr. Anthony Cerami, an authority on the way diabetics' elevated blood-glucose levels damage their bodies, thinks that excess glucose may age you prematurely. Another theory, pooh-poohed by academic medicine, is that a diet high in sugar is the main culprit in *Candida albicans* infections, or dangerous overgrowths of yeast. Such overgrowths have a direct adverse effect on digestion, mainly because they upset the balance of your colonic flora.

Yeasts are a type of fungus, organisms found everywhere in nature, including your large intestine; they are an important part of your intestinal flora. But many twentieth-century habits, among them eating lots of sugar and taking medications like antibiotics, birth control pills, and steroids, can help yeasts flourish—so much so that they begin to dominate your internal ecology, unbalancing it. The results can be a wide range of symptoms, not limited to gastrointestinal upset. Yeasts can cause vaginal infections and urinary disorders, muscle pain, premenstrual difficulties, drowsiness, respiratory problems, depression—to name only a few possibilities. In the previous section on alcohol, I mentioned how alcoholics may incur yeast infections; this is partly because most drinks contain sugar. And then the drinkers unwittingly make these infections worse with sugary coffee and food.

Eating sugar in the form of candies, dairy products, and artificial sweeteners that contain lactose definitely has been corrrelated with vaginal yeast infections. On other fronts, established medicine maintains that there is not enough data to link yeast infections to such a wide variety of symptoms, some of them admittedly vague. The prestigious and influential *Harvard Medical School Health Letter* stated recently that while yeasts' link to illness deserves some attention, "there is no more reason to believe that *Candida* is responsible for an epidemic of chronic disease in otherwise normal people than there ever was to believe that the moon was made of green cheese."

Nevertheless, Dr. C. Orian Truss, the allergist who pioneered treatment for candidal infections and wrote *The Missing Diagnosis*, the first book on yeasts' pernicious influence, points out that the proof of the pudding is in the eating, so to speak: "If you suspect yeast, and treat for it, the treatment works." Truss likens yeast infection to Lyme disease. Its symptoms are so broad that there is no foolproof diagnostic test for it. But Truss says, "Even when test results are equivocal, we know Lyme disease exists because if we apply the right therapy, it clears up."

In the next chapter, when we get into the third week of the Hoffman Program, I'll be highlighting more causes of yeast infections. If you suspect you have one, visit a sympathetic doctor to confirm the diagnosis and provide a nystatin prescription. But your first step is to help yourself by swearing off the sin of extra sugar. Start reading labels carefully, even in health-food stores. Their products are just as liable to be full of honey, molasses, and fructose—watch out for cookies flavored with fruit juice! You'll get all the glucose your body needs from vegetables, grains, and moderate portions of fresh fruit.

Giving up sugar isn't a snap, even if you think you don't have a sweet tooth. If you haven't been paying attention, you've been eating a great deal in disguised forms ever since you were an infant. By now, sugar has become a subtle addiction. Suddenly you may crave it, even if you never consciously did so before. Or you may crave milk more than you ever have—because you want milk sugar. Try eating more complex carbohydrates, especially whole grains and beans. They contain sugar, but release it slowly as you digest, not in a big jolt that encourages fermentation.

The Fifth Sin: Fat. Cut It Down.

In a Buddhist ritual to ensure luck in the new year, Tibetan monks sculpt colored butter into delicate, intricate forms. It's a pretty symbol of fat's essential role in our diet. Fat tastes good, and it's our most filling nutrient. The slow pace at which it moves through your digestive tract leaves you feeling satisfied for longer. Fat carries fat-soluble vitamins like A, D, and E into your bloodstream, and is a crucial source of the fatty acids your gut needs to rebuild its walls.

For modern Westerners, however, fat is no longer good fortune—it's anything but! We need some fat to live, but like sugar, it has crept into our diet in greater and greater proportions.

WHAT'S WRONG WITH FAT?
Well, it depends on what kind you're eating. Too much animal fat is dangerous because it's full of—

• **Cholesterol:** A chemical produced by your liver, it's essential in small amounts for producing hormones and building cells. But excessive amounts end up on your artery walls, eventually clogging them and leading to heart disease. And there's much, much more cholesterol than you need in American favorites like hot dogs, hamburgers, and bacon.

- **Saturated fats:** Your body processes these fatty molecules to increase blood cholesterol levels. Like cholesterol, excess saturated fats are linked to heart disease. Saturated fats crop up in whole milk, ice cream, butter, cheese, and lard. Other major sources are tropical oils like palm, palm kernel, and coconut oil. Palm oil is 51 percent saturated fat, palm kernel oil 88 percent, and coconut oil a whopping 89 percent! Since these products don't come from animals, they don't contain cholesterol, but they do cause your body to produce it.

Our number-one source of fat is meat, especially beef. Nowadays, domestic animals are raised to produce meat that is as well marbled with fat as possible, because it's tenderer and tastes juicier.

What's more, we're surrounded by hidden fat. State meat-labeling laws are so lax that ground beef sold in supermarkets as "lean" actually contains an average of 21 percent fat. Cheese (see table on low-fat cheese in next chapter), whole milk, other dairy products, nondairy creamers, commercial baked goods, and salad dressings also contribute hidden fat to our diet. Nuts and avocados are good sources of important nutrients, but except for chestnuts, they are quite fatty. Another source of hidden fats are the tropical oils, which are worse for your arteries than lard, used as shortening in packaged cookies, crackers, and candies, including health-food varieties. A label that reads "No cholesterol" or "100 percent vegetable shortening" is no guarantee that the product doesn't contain saturated or hydrogenated fat.

KILLER FAT

Fat's greatest danger is its contribution to colon cancer, the second most frequent cancer killer. Every day, your liver secretes bile, a potential carcinogen, into your intestinal tract. Normally bile is diluted and flushed out before it can accumulate and do harm. But a high-fat diet seems to increase the concentration of bile acids in your colon. And unusually high levels of bile may promote tumors. One three-year British study found that patients with colon cancer consumed more foods high in both fat and sugar, like cakes, cookies, and packaged desserts.

Fat is also linked to pancreatic cancer, the fifth leading cause of cancer death in the United States. Like colon cancer, it is prevalent in

Western countries, and may be on the rise. When too much fat—and consequently too much bile—clogs your intestines, some bile may back up into the pancreas. There it may irritate pancreatic tissues and encourage tumors.

Aside from these very dangerous diseases, too much fat can act like a mineral-oil laxative because it overwhelms your ability to digest it. You'd see what I mean if you sat down and ate two whole bars of butter—*not* something I advise trying, by the way. You'd just have to run for the bathroom because you'd have exceeded your absorption threshold.

In the long run, a high-fat diet can interfere with your gut's ability to "talk" to its various parts. Fat is a powerful stimulant of cholecystokinin (CCK), a peptide that is part of your digestive tract's communication system. Overstimulation causes too much peristalsis, and ultimately jams the system with too many signals, guaranteeing digestive trouble.

HOW TO FIGHT BACK

Your keenest weapon against too much fat seems to be fiber. It whisks dangerous carcinogens out of your digestive tract, lessening the danger of colon or pancreatic cancer. Another British study found that while a high-fiber, low-fat diet was better for you, even a high-fat diet that also was 25 percent fiber meant fewer colorectal tumors. And your risk of pancreatic cancer seems to increase if you eat fiberless white bread, but goes down if you consume raw, fiber-rich fruit and vegetables.

But while eating more fiber, remember that fiber alone is no panacea. Protests from consumers worried about cholesterol have prompted some food companies to replace tropical oils in packaged goods with less saturated soybean or cottonseed oil, that pose less risk to your cardiovascular system. But sometimes manufacturers simply add a little oat bran, without removing fat. Or they replace the oils with "artificial" fat—no improvement at all. Artificial saturated fats such as margarine, Crisco, and partially hydrogenated corn oil are so bad for your arteries that if my patients have low cholesterol levels, I urge them to eat butter instead.

And remember that not all animal or vegetable fats are bad for you. Switch to olive oil for cooking and salad dressings. Like the Eskimos and the Finns, eat plenty of fish: fish oil protects your heart and your digestive tract. Instead of fatty beef and pork, buy range-fed poultry and game. Many farm animals are overfed or kept confined in order to increase the ratio of fat to muscles in their meat. Then it is tender, tasty—and full of cholesterol. But free-range animals, who are allowed to move about to graze, produce meat that is akin to game. Some surprising research found that game contains large amounts of more beneficial polyunsaturated fatty acids, like those found in vegetable oils.

The Sixth Sin: Junk Food. Cut It Out.

Many of the diet sins we've been talking about qualify as junk food, including alcohol and coffee. Junk food is low in nutrients and usually high in calories. It is rich in sugar, fat, salt, chemical preservatives, and little else. Comedian Marshall Efron has pointed out that Potato Crisps use chemicals and preservatives—not potatoes—to taste like French fries. And Kool-Aid—"no muss, no fuss, no fresh fruit"—contains so many chemicals that Efron wondered, "What would it do if you put it in a metal pitcher?"

Take the accompanying test called "What's Your Junk-Food Score?" Any score at all is a bad score. We all have some junk-food weakness, even if it's only gum—which is full of artificial sweeteners. And if you checked "Every day" or "Up to 3 times a week" for any item, you're in abysmal dietary shape. No wonder your stomach aches!

Another name for junk food is fast food. It seems to be the gastronomic price we pay for modern times: Speed is becoming a key ingredient of most American meals. In 1989, we spent some $60 billion on fast food. Convenience food, TV dinners, and fast-food franchises mean that we can fill our stomachs quickly, but don't guarantee that we're well fed.

In my experience, if something is worth doing, it takes time. To do anything well, you have to schedule it. And that includes eating well. No question about it: a big part of junk food's attraction is that it's ready to eat—no muss, no fuss, and no nutrients to speak of! If you're devoted to eating the American way, and you want your abdominal trouble to clear up, put eating food that's good for you among your top priorities. Eating right *will* take more time, but if you give up eating fast foods, you won't lose any more time to feeling bad.

WHAT'S YOUR JUNK-FOOD SCORE?

There's no way to win this game: any score means you're losing nutritionally. The point is to become aware of how much junk food you may be eating throughout the day, especially if you "graze" on small amounts all day long, thinking you're eating very little. Exactly how often do you play nutrition roulette by indulging in the following junk foods?

Junk Food	Every day	Up to 3 times a week	Once every 2 weeks	Once a month	Once every 2 months	Never
Instant breakfasts						
Sugary cold cereal						
Processed meats like sausage and bacon						
Soda pop						
Potato chips						
French fries						
Ketchup						
Fast-food burger or cheeseburger						
Cheese spreads						
Fast-food chocolate shake or malted						
Fried chicken						
Puddings and other instant desserts						

If you eat any of the listed foods "Every day," that's way too much. Changing your lousy diet probably will help your digestive problems considerably. Here's why:

• **Instant breakfasts:** Unlike whole grains and fiber, these contain sugar and refined carbohydrates.

(continued on page 70)

(continued from page 69)

• **Sugary cold cereal:** In most cases, these are just as bad as instant breakfasts. Remember back in the early 1970s, when Congress held hearings on the content of cold cereals? In some cases, legislators discovered, you were better off eating the box!

• **Processed meats:** Sausage and bacon taste great with eggs; cold cuts make good sandwiches. But they all contain preservatives, mostly nitrates and nitrites.

• **Soda pop:** It contains plenty of sugar and often caffeine as well.

• **Potato chips and French fries:** An unadorned potato is a fine carbohydrate, low in calories and quite rich in vitamin B. Once fried, however, it's high only in fat and calories.

• **Ketchup:** Before you wax nostalgic for the Reagan era, when ketchup was a vegetable, remember that most commercial seasonings are full of sugar, artificial flavorings, and preservatives.

• **Burger or cheeseburger:** The Center for Science in the Public Interest has rated these fast foods highest in fat.

• **Cheese spreads:** Lots of fat, preservatives, and artificial flavoring.

• **Chocolate shake or malted:** According to the Center for Science in the Public Interest, these fast foods are highest in sugar. Chocolate contains caffeine, and maltose is another form of sugar.

• **Fried chicken:** Usually very high in fat and cholesterol. Some fast-food chains are beginning to use natural vegetable oils for frying, rather than oils high in saturated animal or vegetable fat. And some are introducing roast chicken—sometimes even range-fed birds.

• **Instant desserts:** More sugar and empty carbohydrates.

The Seventh Sin: Antacids. Cut Them Out.

"Wait a minute!" I bet you're saying. "My stomach *hurts*. When I take antacids, it feels *better*. Why are you telling me to give up *medication*?"

First of all, if you've successfully eliminated or cut down on the other six Deadly Diet Sins, you may not need antacids anymore. Your trouble probably wasn't too much stomach acid, but eating the wrong foods or overeating.

Secondly, most antacids have been proven useless. In a Swedish experiment published in 1986, patients with chronic upset stomachs but no sign of ulcers were given either placebos or over-the-counter antacids. These two groups of people with stomach pain improved at exactly the same rate, a measly 4 percent. In short, antacids won't help your upset stomach much.

More evidence against antacids comes from the Public Citizen Health Research Group, a Ralph Nader organization that published a study of over-the-counter medicines. While antacids could help heartburn, "most upset stomachs," the group concluded, "are not the result of too much acid and need not be treated with antacids." The group could not recommend Alka-Seltzer, a popular antacid, even though the FDA has approved all its ingredients. According to the group, the problem was that all these ingredients are ineffective. Aspirin can actually irritate your gut.

The main reason antacids don't work is that while you take them to offset too much stomach acid, they actually give you more. This is called "acid rebound." In reaction to your medicine, your stomach produces even more acid, so that you end up feeling worse than ever. Then you pour *another* dose of antacid down your gut, and the cycle continues.

ANTACIDS ARE NOT ONLY USELESS, THEY CAN
HURT YOU

Your digestive tract may also become too alkaline, thanks to antacid. Then you become vulnerable to nasty microbes that your stomach acid had held in check. Since gastric acid helps you absorb nutrients like iron and calcium, you also may become prey to anemia or osteoporosis. And too much antacid disrupts the balance of your colonic flora, exposing you to more very serious infections.

When you take antacids for a prolonged period, your kidneys have to work overtime to excrete the excess alkali your medicine has flooded into your gut. So antacids can predispose you to kidney stones and some types of urinary tract infections. If you're taking other medicine as well, your kidneys may have trouble processing those drugs.

Here are some common antacid ingredients that do you no good at all:

• *Calcium carbonate:* It comes from chalk, the first antacid people tried. Calcium carbonate still tastes chalky. The main ingredient in Tums, it is also constipating, sometimes severely. If you combine a good deal of milk or other dairy products with daily doses of calcium carbonate, as doctors encouraged people to do in the early days of ulcer treatment, your system can overdose on calcium. Then you may develop not only kidney stones but calcification of the kidneys, one step away from kidney failure.

• *Sodium bicarbonate:* Like calcium carbonate, sodium bicarbonate, especially if combined with milk, can make your gastrointestinal system much too alkaline and harm your kidneys. The sodium in this antacid can also cause high blood pressure.

• *Magnesium hydroxide:* The main ingredient in milk of magnesia, it doesn't cause much acid rebound, but it can clean you out! To prevent diarrhea, you have to alternate it with a constipating antacid.

• *Aluminum hydroxide:* Because it particularly depletes phosphorus, it may thin your bones and waste your muscles. And it causes constipation.

THE ALUMINUM-ANTACID CONNECTION

Another risk in taking antacids is that most popular brands, including Gelusil, Maalox, and Mylanta, contain aluminum, a toxic metal that has been implicated in Alzheimer's disease, pulmonary and bone disease, as well as heart trouble and anemia in kidney patients. In normal people, aluminum slows stomach and intestinal muscle contractions. This delays your stomach's emptying into your intestines, and contributes to constipation.

Normally, your bodily levels of aluminum are very low. But according to Dr. Michael A. Weiner, who has studied aluminum's noxious effects, people who take large amounts of antacids can add over 160 times more aluminum to their systems per day! Aluminum also shows up in food additives, including some in cake mixes, frozen dough, self-rising flour, processed cheese, and baking powder.

BEYOND ANTACIDS

"Fine!" you say, "your evidence is pretty convincing, doctor. But what do I do the next time my stomach aches?" Most upset stomachs are a reaction to stress or to the wrong food. Time and relaxation are the best healers, so take a break and clear your medicine cabinet of antacids. Stock up on aloe vera gel—stronger than so-called aloe vera juice, which is actually gel diluted with water. Aloe vera tastes bitter, but it soothes and heals your gut rapidly and safely. And keep reading! In the next five weeks of the Hoffman Program, you'll pick up many more new stomach strategies.

Weeks Three
and Four:
Play Diet Detective

"I don't like stories about arsenic in food."

—*Nero Wolfe, the oversized gourmand-detective,*
in Too Many Cooks, *by Rex Stout*

Perhaps you haven't been committing any of the Seven Deadly
Diet Sins. You're well informed about nutrition, and make an effort to
stay away from sugar, fat, and packaged goods. Why, then, are you
still having stomach problems?

All the healthful habits in the world are no help if your body is
reacting as if your food were poison. In other words, perhaps you're
allergic to what you're eating, or you have a food intolerance, that is,
an inability to digest certain things properly.

Food allergies can strike anyone, for no reason at all, though you
may be more prone if there's a history of allergy in your family, or if
you already have signs of allergy, such as asthma or eczema. At least
one of every six Americans, roughly 40 million people, suffers from
asthma or some other allergic disease. Like other kinds of allergy—to
animals, pollen, or dust—food allergies are not diseases but symptoms. They're actually a normal bodily response gone awry—signs that
your immune system cannot distinguish a nutrient from something
toxic in your environment. Consequently, your immune system mis-

takenly launches an attack to destroy the nutrient. You experience this attack as classic allergic symptoms: sneezing, asthma, runny nose, headache, skin irritations like eczema or acne—or stomach pain.

If you are allergic, as many people are, to casein, a protein in dairy products, you have a true allergy. Bad reactions to certain foods—for example, sugar and coffee—are not allergies but food intolerances. These are bodily reactions that may be psychological (you just can't abide a certain food), physiological (there's a physical reason why you react a particular way), or pharmacological (the food has a druglike effect on your body). Many signs of food intolerance are the same as allergic reactions. However, whatever reaction you have does *not* involve your immune system.

Medical researchers know much more about allergies than they do about food intolerances. Some foods—spices, for instance—may irritate your gut because it's already diseased. Other food intolerances can be very idiosyncratic; you may never meet anyone else who has your particular sensitivity or personal food reactions. One reason you may not be able to tolerate a certain food is that it's hard to break down anyway, or you lack the enzyme necessary to digest it properly. If you can't drink milk, for example, without suffering indigestion or diarrhea, you're deficient in lactase, the enzyme that helps your gut digest lactose, or milk sugar.

I think that there probably is a very good reason that many of us cannot tolerate grains or dairy products: we haven't evolved to do so. Millions of years ago in prehistory, when our digestive system was evolving, there were no domesticated animals, and hence no dairy products. Grains are also a relatively modern food; they were unavailable except in small quantities until people started farming. And now consider the vast amounts of grain you eat today—from breakfast cereal to pasta dinner. Some of it is disguised, like the corn in corn syrup or cornstarch in your last Chinese meal. So if you cannot tolerate grains, you may be at risk more frequently than you realize.

Food allergies or intolerances may be at the root of some serious gastrointestinal problems like colitis and some chronic illnesses like irritable bowel syndrome. (I'll be talking more about both problems in Part Three of this book.) Such sensitivities also may cause minor but uncomfortable conditions like nausea, indigestion, vomiting, bad breath, painful bloating and gas, diarrhea, constipation, cramping. But since antibodies to allergens are found all over your body, you may feel symptoms anywhere, not just in your digestive tract. In fact, inability to tolerate gluten, a protein found in many grains, can have widespread effects on your body. It can even bring on diseases of the immune system itself, known as autoimmune diseases. Food allergies also can be mistaken for other sorts of allergies or illnesses. And like other allergies, food allergies or intolerances can alter your mood or cause psychological symptoms like depression or anxiety.

Your Doctor Plays Detective

Not surprisingly, then, food intolerances are notoriously difficult to diagnose, much more so than allergies to animals, plants, dust, or molds. Some people cannot tolerate ingredients that are widely used and not necessarily obvious, like corn, milk, eggs, wheat, and certain spices. And food intolerances don't play fair. You may not be able to tolerate something nutritious—milk, eggs, tomatoes, or apples, to name only a few possibilities. Or you may be intolerant to your favorite foods, the ones you crave most often. Whenever I suspect food intolerance, I usually start by asking patients to name their favorite treats. One woman listed chocolate, fish, raspberries, whipped cream, and champagne. When I tested her we discovered, to her chagrin, that only fish was safe for her.

For any food intolerance test, you will have to see an allergist or a nutritionally oriented physician. There are some special tests for particular problems, like the breath test for lactose intolerance. As part of this test, you put a mask over your mouth and breathe into a machine which measures the amount of hydrogen in your breath. Excessive hydrogen is a clue that you're not digesting lactose, or milk sugar, properly.

Many food intolerances don't show up on standard blood tests for allergies or even skin tests. In a skin test, the doctor injects under your skin a little bit of the food you suspect is the cause of your discomfort. If you almost immediately see whealing (raised, reddened patches on your skin) or feel a systemic reaction like mental fogginess, then you have found the offending food. Most food sensitivities, however, combine an immediate reaction—nausea, for instance—with delayed ones like cramps, headaches, fatigue, runny nose, itching, or mental problems that develop hours or even days after you've consumed an offending substance. Skin tests can't link these late-blooming symptoms to a certain food.

Like skin tests, conventional blood tests for allergies measure mostly immediate sensitivities and miss delayed ones. Some blood tests only link foods with obvious, life-threatening reactions, like choking, which can happen if you are allergic to nuts. Blood tests also can be much too general to detect your own peculiar food sensitivities. It's not unusual to take a blood test and get results that show you are allergic to twenty or thirty foods! People who for religious reasons have never touched pork once in their entire lives have been told that they are allergic to it—a physical impossibility.

Blood tests may yield completely misleading results because they're measuring a lot of physiological static in your body that has nothing to do with reactions to food. I've had better luck with a blood test called IgG4, which measures only one particular subset of long-term allergic reactions, and therefore doesn't exaggerate or, conversely, underestimate allergic reactions.

When skin and blood tests do work, they can provide a shortcut detection method. But most of them are very limited. The trouble is they rely on your body's immunological memory. They check what happens at the surface of your skin when a certain food enters your body, or whether your blood "remembers" being allergic to this substance. But they cannot measure what happens when the rubber meets the road—that is, when a particular food enters your digestive tract. There you may have a totally unpredictable reaction—which happens so long after you've eaten that you may never suspect that a particular food is the culprit. And, of course, your reaction actually may reflect food intolerance rather than true allergy—for instance, intestinal bloating (a common reaction to sugar), diarrhea (due to apple juice), or cramping (commonly caused by caffeine).

Playing Detective Yourself

In the end, food intolerances are one stomach problem that you truly are better off diagnosing and treating yourself. Treatment is very simple: stop eating foods that affect you badly!

To play diet detective and figure out what your problem foods are, you need only two tools in your detection kit: your food diary and one

---

very simple diet, the Hoffman Pain-Stopper Diet. By following my special diet, you can pinpoint any food or family of foods that might be upsetting your stomach. For each food, you'll need two weeks on this diet: one week to lay off the food in question, plus one more week to start eating it again and watch what happens. Even children can follow my plan: if yours are too young to keep a personal diary, you can do it for them.

First of all, before you start thinking about the diet itself, go back over your food diary. I hope that you've been updating it *every day*. Trying to reconstruct Thursday's meals and moods when you finally find the time on Saturday morning is practically useless. Because allergic reactions are often delayed and subtle, you *must* be conscientious about writing down what you've eaten and how you felt afterward, physically and emotionally.

As you retrace your meals, take a highlighter and mark the times when you had stomach pain. If you had cramps one evening, look up what you ate at your most recent meal, and also 24 or even 36 hours earlier. Here's where you need to start doing detective work: because your digestive tract can take that long to completely pass food, allergies may not affect you until a few days or even a week later. If you backtrack your food intake, you may be able to at least narrow down your possible problem foods to a few suspects. Once you've done so, you have a good chance of finding the food or foods that are the roots of your symptoms by means of my special Pain-Stopper Diet, which I'll explain shortly.

Meanwhile, as you go over your diary, pay as close attention as Nero Wolfe, the famous detective and fussy eater, gave to every single meal. List your favorite foods and—painful as the thought of doing without them may be—check what happened after you ate them. Is that bowl of Wheaties or warm corn muffin that seems like the only reason to get up every morning really making you ill? After your favorites, consider carefully the following six brands of food criminals: they're the usual suspects in food allergy cases.

Suspect Number One: A Big Clue—It Comes From Cows

If you are sensitive to milk and other dairy products, you may have lactose intolerance, or allergies to ingredients in these foods. There are

THE MOST VICIOUS FOOD OFFENDERS

A trip down the digestive tract—with plenty of potholes. Here are the foods most likely to provoke symptoms in anyone with food allergies or intolerances, and exactly where you can expect to feel discomfort.

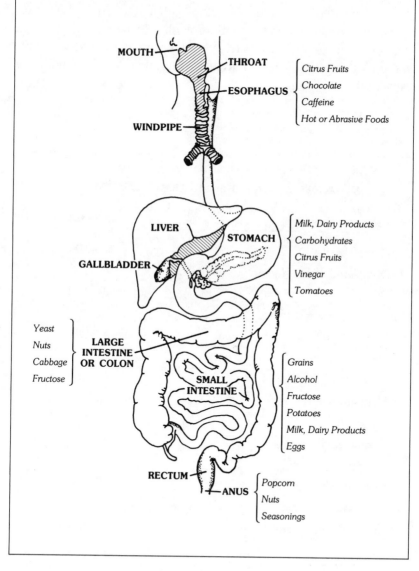

actually three different ways milk and dairy products can upset digestion, but you can be affected by two or even all three simultaneously. The only effective way to treat any of the three is to figure out your own level of tolerance and adjust your diet accordingly; there is no allergy medicine that will suppress your symptoms.

• *Lactose Intolerance:* The first won't show up on an allergy test, because it is a sensitivity, not a true allergy. Lactose intolerance is likely to affect you if you are a black or Oriental adult. It also affects some Latin American and Caribbean adults, as well as whites from Mediterranean countries. It rarely shows up in children or in people whose roots are in northern Europe or central Asia, where milk is a staple in the local diet.

INCIDENCE OF LACTOSE INTOLERANCE IN ADULTS

Ethnic Group	% Intolerant
African blacks	97–100
Dravidian Indians (India)	95–100
Orientals	90–100
North American Indians	80–90
Central/South American Indians	70–90
Mexican Americans	70–80
North American blacks	70–75
Mediterraneans	60–90
Jews	60–80
Central & Northern Indians (India)	25–65
Middle Europeans	10–20
North American whites	7–15
Northwestern Indians (India/Pakistan)	3–15
Northern Europeans	1–5

WHICH FOODS CONTAIN LACTOSE?

Product	Unit	Lactose (approx. grams/unit)
MILK	1 cup (244 grams)	11
Low-fat milk, 2% fat	1 cup (244 grams)	9–13
Skim milk	1 cup (244 grams)	12–14
Chocolate milk	1 cup (244 grams)	10–12
Sweetened condensed whole milk	1 cup (306 grams)	35
Dried whole milk	1 cup (128 grams)	48
Nonfat dry milk instant	1½ cups (128 grams)	46
Buttermilk fluid	1 cup (245 grams)	9–11
Whipped cream topping	1 tablespoon (3 grams)	0.4
Light cream	1 tablespoon (15 grams)	0.6
Half and Half	1 tablespoon (15 grams)	0.6
CHEESE:		
Blue	1 oz. (28 grams)	0.7
*Camembert	1 oz. (28 grams)	0.1
*Cheddar	1 oz. (28 grams)	0.4–0.6
Colby	1 oz. (28 grams)	0.7
Cream	1 oz. (28 grams)	0.8
Gouda	1 oz. (28 grams)	0.6
Parmesan, grated	1 oz. (28 grams)	0.8
*American (processed)	1 oz. (28 grams)	0.5

(continued on page 82)

(continued from page 81)

*Swiss	1 oz. (28 grams)	0.4–0.6
Cottage cheese	1 cup (210 grams)	5–6
Cottage cheese, low-fat, 2% fat	1 cup (226 grams)	7–8
BUTTER	2 pats (10 grams)	0.1
OLEOMARGARINE	2 pats (10 grams)	0
ICE CREAM:		
Vanilla, regular	1 cup (133 grams)	9
Ice milk, vanilla	1 cup (131 grams)	10

Other foods containing small but significant amounts of lactose are nondairy coffee creamers, some fats, liqueurs and cordials, breaded chicken, liverwurst and frankfurters, many candies, and milk-based infant formulas.
* Some cheeses are almost lactose-free: brick, Camembert, Cheddar, Edam, provolone, Swiss, American.

Source: From *Diet Therapy in Adult Lactose Malabsorption: Present Practices*, by Jack D. Welsh, M.D., *American Journal of Clinical Nutrition*, Volume 31, April 1978, pages 592–96.

If you cannot tolerate lactose, most likely you react badly to milk and ice cream, but not to most cheeses or yogurt, cultured milk products in which fermentation has digested much of the lactose for you. To cope with your intolerance, you either can avoid unfermented dairy products or, if you like eating them, can use Lactaid to help you digest them.

Lactaid milk is a low-fat milk treated with lactase, the very enzyme you lack. Available in most supermarkets, Lactaid milk is about one-third more expensive than regular milk. It tastes slightly sweeter and contains 70 to 85 percent less lactose. The same company also makes fat-free Lactaid skim milk and CalciMilk, a low-fat, lactose-reduced milk with about two-thirds more calcium than other low-fat milks.

If you prefer to treat your own milk to cut lactose, you can buy Lactaid drops. You have to wait 24 hours for the drops in milk to take effect, but five drops per quart reduces milk sugar by about 70 percent. This method is a little cheaper, and has little effect on the taste of the milk. If you want to indulge yourself with ice cream or some other dairy product for which there's no lactose-reduced substitute, take Lactaid enzyme tablets (sold over the counter in most drugstores) just before your meal.

I've already mentioned that chocolate, which contains caffeine, can be a culprit in cases of gastritis and heartburn. But strangely enough, if you have trouble digesting lactose, you *may* be able to enjoy a nice soothing cup of hot milky cocoa—which even sounds as though it would settle your stomach. Despite chocolate's bad reputation as far as indigestion and heartburn are concerned, there's some evidence that it can help you digest milk. That's probably because chocolate, like coffee and grapefruit, is one of the few bitter foods we eat, and all of them are, at least in part, digestive aids.

• *Allergy to Milk Protein:* An allergy test can reveal another possibility: you may be allergic to one or more of the proteins in milk. In that case, you'll feel off-color if you drink milk—or eat yogurt, cheese, or anything else made with milk, including Lactaid or treated milk. You simply must avoid all milk and milk products.

• *Fat Intolerance:* Finally, because of a pancreatic insufficiency, you may be unable to tolerate fats in general, not just milk fats. This intolerance won't show up on an allergy test, but if fats are your digestive deviation, you'll tend to feel an urgent need to defecate soon after meals. You'll have diarrhea or loose stools and bloating. You'll react especially strongly to rich dairy products like heavy cream, sour cream, crème fraîche, whole milk, butter, and gourmet ice cream. (Häagen-Dazs, sadly, is particularly high in fat.) You may not be as sensitive to skim milk or low-fat cheese. If you want dairy protein and calcium without deleterious fat, stick to skim milk, which is virtually fat-free. Whole milk is 4 percent fat, and milk that is 1 or 2 percent fat may also give you trouble.

Among other alternatives, ice milk is less fatty than ice cream, but it still contains a generous portion of fat. And as you can see from the accompanying chart, there's almost no such thing as low-fat cheese. Try spreading part-skim ricotta on bread instead of cream cheese or butter. Choose mozzarella made from buffalo milk, yogurt, low-fat cottage cheese, and chèvre, or goat cheese. Both buffalo and goat's milk are much less fatty than cow's milk.

SO MUCH FOR LOW-FAT CHEESE!

Cheese is a good source of calcium, riboflavin, and protein, but contains a lot of fat, mostly saturated fat. Anything with more than 7 grams of fat per ounce is a high-fat cheese. Medium-fat is 5 to 7 grams per ounce (feta, part-skim mozzarella). Low-fat is 4 grams or less (farmer's cheese, low-fat ricotta, and Dr. Nathan Pritikin's favorite, sapsago). There's almost no such thing as "low-fat" cheese. Even those made with part skim milk are higher in fat than other sources of calcium or protein.

1 oz. Cheese	Calories	Grams of Protein	of Fat	% Fat
Feta	75	4	6	72
Brie	95	5.9	7.9	75
Cheddar	114	7.1	9.4	74
Gouda	101	7.1	7.8	70
Gruyere	117	8.5	9.2	71
Monterey Jack	106	6.9	8.6	73
Mozzarella	90	6.1	7.0	70
Part-Skim Mozzarella	79	7.8	4.9	56
Muenster	104	6.6	8.5	74
Neufchatel	74	2.8	6.6	80
Parmesan	111	10.1	7.3	60
Grated Parm., 1 Tbsp.	35	2.1	1.5	40
¼ cup Ricotta	108	7	8	67
Part-Skim Ricotta	85	7	5	52
Swiss	96	6.9	7.4	69

Perhaps you have only a partial form of lactose intolerance: sometimes you have symptoms; sometimes you don't. Ice cream gives you the runs, but nothing goes awry if you take milk in your tea. If you have this sort of fifty-fifty reaction, or if you have the first or the third type of dairy sensitivity, you are able to eat yogurt, kefir, some cheeses and—surprise!—buttermilk because they contain a kind of natural Lactaid. Since you can't digest these foods, which are made from milk, by yourself, the beneficial bacteria in them—the ones that changed milk into these milk products in the first place—digest it for you. These live cultures are called lactobacilli. One lactobacilli researcher, Dr. Khem Shahani, has used them to treat lactose intolerance. Some strains, including *Lactobacillus acidophilus,* produce a number of natural antibiotics, and are among the friendly flora that inhabit your colon and help you digest. If you don't like yogurt or other milk products, taking lactobacilli or acidophilus supplements can help populate your gastric tract with lactose-digesting bacteria. Pass up sweet acidophilus milk, however; it contains just as much lactose as regular milk.

Perhaps you're concerned about getting enough calcium because your lactose intolerance forces you to avoid most dairy products. In the next week of the Hoffman Program, I'll be telling you how to get plenty of calcium in other ways.

Suspect Number Two: A Big Clue—Tastes Too Good to Be Bad

During Weeks One and Two of the Hoffman Program, you kicked your sugar habit. Your sucrose habit, that is. Sucrose is only one of sugar's several forms. Lactose, or milk sugar, is another one, and it can give you digestive trouble. A third form is fructose, found in all fruits and some vegetables, like corn. Just because fructose is found in nature, that doesn't necessarily mean you can digest it comfortably.

Perhaps you crave fruits because they're so sweet—but then your favorites cause you pain. Fructose may be the reason. If you can't wait for strawberry season, try skipping it this year; you might feel better. Fructose can cause indigestion because it takes a relatively long time to digest. In fact, 71 percent of all adults cannot completely absorb it. When you think about it, this is not all that surprising. The fruits we enjoy today really aren't all that "natural." Thanks to modern agricultural expertise, they are much more succulent and many times sweeter than their ancestors, which prehistoric people occasionally plucked in season from trees and bushes in the wild. For cavemen, fruits were a rare treat; now they're plentiful all year round, flown into our markets from Chile or New Zealand. Dried fruits and fruit juice, particularly blended varieties, which can be especially hard on your gut, were nonexistent in the Stone Age.

Not everyone who is sensitive to fructose is terribly uncomfortable after eating a piece of fruit or drinking juice or soft drinks, many of which are sweetened with high-fructose corn syrup. But if you are susceptible to fructose, you may have cramps or osmotic diarrhea—the kind you're apt to describe as "my meals just run right through me." What actually happens is that when a big load of fructose hits your stomach after you eat an apple or drink a can of soda, the fructose pulls extra water into your gut. Then food passes through very quickly—too quickly to feel comfortable. Some people who suffer from irritable bowel syndrome have found relief on a fructose-free diet. They really may have been suffering from fructose intolerance all along.

Regardless of the old saw about "an apple a day," apples are prime offenders in stomachs that are sensitive to fructose. Even organically grown apples can affect you for the worse. Most foods that naturally contain fructose—for example, fruits and honey—have about equal amounts of fructose and glucose, another, less irritating form of sugar. However, apples and apple juice contain three times as much fructose as glucose. The same is true of foods to which apple juice or concentrate has been added as a sweetener. You may be unable to tolerate apples, and apple juice may be giving your baby diarrhea.

Another potential pitfall are the new health-food cookies, preserves, and other goodies that advertise themselves as "sugar-free" because they are flavored with honey or fruit juices, frequently apple concentrate. If you have given up sugar but hoped you could still enjoy these "healthy" desserts, look out! These treats are certainly delicious—some much more so than standard supermarket products—but if you are sensitive to fructose, your digestive tract will have to pay.

You may be worried that if you give up fruit, you won't get enough vitamin C. Actually, you can get plenty of this nutrient from vegetables, especially red peppers, broccoli, and cabbage. The National Center for Health Statistics has found that 40 percent of U.S. adults do not eat a single fruit on a given day. Those hundred million fruit-dodging Americans aren't necessarily courting nutritional disaster—provided they are not also doing without vegetables.

Suspect Number Three: A Big Clue—You Feel Worse After the Movies

You may not be able to tolerate some foods because they are simply too abrasive to pass through your digestive tract comfortably. Many of these foods may be your special favorites: popcorn, whole nuts and seeds (but thankfully, *not* nut butters—although, as you'll learn in the next section, they may upset your stomach because they cause gas). Other troublemakers are apple peel and other fruit skins, berries and similar fruits with lots of seeds—strawberries, raspberries, blackberries, gooseberries. All of these foods contain fiber, and normally the more fibrous foods you eat, the better. But these foods can overload your system with roughage and give you diarrhea or cause you pain.

Suspect Number Four:
A Big Clue—A Big Toot

Another source of potential food intolerance is foods that produce a great deal of gas. You know the ditty—

> Baked beans,
> The musical fruit—
> The more you eat,
> The more you toot!

Even a waitress in a Hemingway novel quotes these lines.

People who have trouble with abrasive foods usually can eat nut butters, but those who cannot tolerate gas-forming foods have to pass up peanut butter or cashew butter sandwiches. If you can't tolerate nuts, beans, fruit, and other gassy foods, the reason is that they either are completely indigestible or contain ingredients that are indigestible or relatively hard to break down in your stomach. Seeds fall into the first category: they resist digestion—a fact that ensures the survival of plant and tree species. Once a fruit or vegetable is eaten by an animal, the seeds can travel in its stomach far from their parent tree or bush. When the animal defecates, the seeds, still intact, can start growing in new ground.

Beans, Hemingway's favorite, and other legumes contain oligosaccharides, long chains of sugars which you cannot break down in your small intestine because you have no enzymes that will do so. So, when these sugars move into the lower intestine, bacteria feed on them to produce gases made of carbon dioxide, hydrogen, and methane.

Other foods can cause gas and bloating because they have hard-to-digest ingredients. Fruits contain fructose, and nuts and beans contain disaccharides or starch blockers, substances that prevent your body

---

from digesting starches in food. Hence, if you cannot tolerate nuts and fruits, they can give you a bad case of diarrhea. Onions and mushrooms may also give you trouble. For a more detailed discussion of gas problems, see Chapter 8.

Suspect Number Five: A Big Clue—Those "Amber Waves of Grain"

Gluten is a protein found in wheat, barley, rye, oats, and other grains. Scientists aren't sure whether gluten sensitivity is an allergy or a food intolerance, although some people are allergic to wheat, a condition that an allergy test can detect. Gluten sensitivity, on the other hand, is very hard to spot with a test. Signs of gluten sensitivity run the gamut from minor to dangerously severe. Some symptoms are annoying but relatively mild: they include asthma, eczema, and a runny nose. But gluten intolerance also may lie behind some very serious digestive diseases.

Because gluten intolerance causes such a complex range of symptoms, it can be very hard to diagnose. Many people may not realize they have a mild or even severe form; they think their symptoms mean another, entirely different illness. Both wheat allergy and gluten intolerance can mimic irritable bowel syndrome. Or perhaps you have just a *forme fruste*, or tendency toward gluten intolerance, so you have a minor ache here, a little pain there. Understandably, your doctor may attribute your symptoms to any number of causes and completely overlook the fact that a food triggers your troubles.

THE WORST CASES

In its severest forms, gluten intolerance can lead to inflammatory bowel disease, which I'll be discussing later, and celiac sprue, or celiac disease. Medical researchers discovered celiac sprue about a hundred years ago, when one investigator noticed that certain children who grew poorly also ate quantities of bread. Conversely, when bread was eliminated from their diet, their normal growth resumed. The exact cause of celiac disease may be a combination of gluten intolerance with genetic predisposition and a particular virus. Its digestive consequences are very clear: it destroys millions of villi, the threadlike projections that line the folds of the inner lining of your small intestine and give it a velvety appearance. In some celiac sprue patients, so many villi have been damaged that the small intestine's lining looks flat, not folded. Once injured, villi can't do their job properly: they can't transfer nutrients into your blood so they can be distributed to cells throughout your body.

This condition, called malabsorption, means that, basically, you remain undernourished no matter how much you eat. That's why the patients who first helped doctors pinpoint gluten intolerance as the cause of celiac sprue had not grown; they were starving on their supposedly nutritious diet of wheat bread.

If you have celiac sprue, malabsorption is so severe that it is threatening your life. To some degree, however, malabsorption accompanies every single type of digestive disorder. A key sign of malabsorption—one that you can easily spot for yourself—is fatty diarrhea. You have loose, voluminous stools, and instead of being processed into your body, fat ends up as an oil slick on the surface of the water in your toilet bowl. Don't mistake the slick for mucus, which usually sinks. This kind of diarrhea accompanies many digestive disorders, but especially celiac sprue. If that's what ails you, you will also have other classic signs of malnutrition like stunted growth in children, emaciation, and even a distended belly, familiar from photos of starving Saharan peoples.

THE BEST MEDICINE

Most of the time, particularly in mild forms, gluten intolerance can masquerade as other, unrelated medical problems. Like fructuse intolerance, it can pass for irritable bowel syndrome. In fact, gluten intolerance is such a good mimic that the only reliable way to detect it is to stop eating gluten. Gluten is found in whole grains like wheat, oats, rye, and barley—but not in corn or buckwheat, despite its name. However, like sugar, gluten sneaks into your diet in many foods—bread, crackers, pasta, doughnuts, cookies, pizza, pancakes, malted milk, pretzels, breaded meat or fish, gravy, desserts made from commercial mixes, cheese spreads, and salad dressings which use wheat as a stabilizer—and even some medications. If you suspect that you're sensitive to gluten, avoid grains and read all food and medicine labels carefully.

Especially if you have celiac disease, your intestinal mucosa is very sensitive even to tiny amounts of gluten in your diet. Researchers in

Pavia, Italy, have reported that this is a particular problem for Catholic school children with celiac disease, who take communion frequently. These young patients would serve their religion and their health better if, despite their tender age, they drank wine: "According to the New Testament," the Italian researchers write, "a wheat-free Host is unacceptable, but it might be theologically acceptable for patients with celiac disease to take holy communion in the form of Christ's blood (consecrated wine) instead of His body."

LIFE BEYOND GLUTEN

Once you purge your diet of gluten, your symptoms quickly disappear. Children who have gluten intolerance frequently outgrow it. But if you have had celiac sprue, your damaged villi will need months to repair themselves, and you will feel run-down for quite some time. Be sure to take vitamin and mineral supplements to make up your deficiencies.

If you cannot digest gluten properly, there are still many foods you can enjoy—even some grains and flours. Safe bets include buckwheat (despite its name—you may know it as kasha), rice, and millet, as well as soybean, chickpea and potato flour. Some health-food stores carry gluten-free pastas. Another wonderful substitute is quinoa (pronounced KEEN-wa), a South American grain that makes an extremely fine, silky flour. A recent book, *Quinoa: The Super Grain* (Briarcliff Manor, New York: Japan Publications, 1988) includes recipes and tips on cooking with quinoa.

Suspect Number Six: A Big Clue—Is the Compost Heap in Your Stomach Out of Control?

Yeasts are living organisms found all over—in foods, in the air, in damp or moldy places—and inside you. They live in your throat, vagina, and other mucous membranes throughout your body, and they are part of the beneficent flora that thrive in your colon and complete the digestive process.

However, yeasts can spread so much that they overwhelm the other flora in your body and unbalance your inner ecology. Especially if you already have a yeast overgrowth, basically a yeast infection, you also may be allergic to yeast, or *Candida albicans*. In fact, an allergist,

Dr. C. Orian Truss, was the first to finger yeast as the prime suspect behind a wide range of allergic reactions. Immunologist Alan Levin of the University of California at San Francisco estimates that one third of all Americans may be prey to *Candida* allergies.

You may be familiar with some of your body's responses to yeast overgrowth: urinary tract and vaginal infections and thrush, a throat infection common in newborns that involves a harmless but aggravating white coating of the tongue. However, you may not recognize stomach troubles like bloating, diarrhea, constipation, heartburn, and indigestion as signs of yeast allergy. Eating certain foods can trigger these painful reactions or a wide range of nondigestive difficulties like acne, migraines, respiratory problems, premenstrual tension, and psychological difficulties such as lethargy, depression, and anxiety.

HIGH ON *CANDIDA*

Have you ever seen birds swooping erratically or flying at a tilt? They've been eating chokeberries that have fermented on their bushes. The same thing may happen to you if you have a *Candida* overgrowth. After all, yeast ferments grapes, potatoes, and grains into alcohol—and it can do the job in your stomach just as well as in a wine barrel or a beer keg. If you feel stoned when you haven't been drinking—especially after a high-carbohydrate meal, like a bowl of pasta—too much *Candida* may be turning your insides into a brewery.

ANTI-*CANDIDA* THERAPY

Like other allergies, *Candida* allergies can be treated. Some sufferers with extreme cases may have to rid their homes of chemical products that can exacerbate their symptoms. Such culprits include cosmetics, household cleaners, chlorinated water—which means that tap water can be hazardous—moth balls, and even synthetic textiles whose chemical ingredients may tax your already overburdened immune system. If you suspect you have a yeast infection, see your doctor for a

---

test and a prescription for nystatin, which suppresses yeast growth. Nystatin is one of the least toxic prescription drugs—safer than most over-the-counter products. The powder form is most effective and least likely to cause adverse reactions. It merely coats the lining of your mouth, pharynx, esophagus, stomach and intestine, preventing yeast from multiplying. Take it after meals and at bedtime, and don't put anything in your mouth for about twenty minutes afterward. That way, a coating of nystatin can cover tissues in your mouth and upper digestive tract.

Most of the time, however, nystatin isn't necessary. Eliminating medicine and foods that encourage yeast growth is enough. Some drugs, including antibiotics, kill off bacteria that normally keep yeast in check. Cortisone reduces your body's defenses against *Candida,* and birth control pills stimulate yeast growth. If you ever have taken any of these drugs for more than two weeks, they may have allowed yeast to spread, so that you have a leftover infection. Acidophilus capsules, available over the counter in most pharmacies and health-food stores, will help clear it up. They also will keep your internal ecology properly balanced whenever you're obliged to take these drugs. If you have a leftover infection, you should also take yeast-free vitamin/mineral supplements to build up immunity.

ANTI-*CANDIDA* DIET

Perhaps your problem is not so much a food intolerance as it is the yeast that certain foods help to grow out of bounds. As I've already mentioned, sugar is the worst culprit. But there are others, including foods that contain simple carbohydrates—dairy products, fruits and fruit juices. Some people do fine if they stick to whole grains and complex carbohydrates; others feel better if they eliminate all grains from their meals, and minimize carbohydrates.

Particularly if you already have a yeast infection, a food allergy test will show that you're sensitive to brewer's or baker's yeast. Even small amounts of foods that already contain yeasts—especially alcoholic beverages, most of which are also full of sugar—can intoxicate you, and feed your personal fungus at the same time. Since this is Week Three of the Hoffman Program, I hope you've already cut out chocolate, colas, and other sugary junk foods.

MIND YOUR MEAT

You should also consider vegetarianism, or at least start choosing only organic, free-range meat and poultry. In the past thirty years, the way most American livestock is bred for meat has changed dramatically. Most farm animals eat feed drenched with insecticides and are injected with antibiotics to stave off illnesses. Often they're also given hormones so that they'll grow and reproduce more rapidly. When you eat a pork chop or a slice of roast beef, the consequences of all this animal doctoring are probably negligible. Certain additives, if used judiciously, certainly do result in healthier animals and more nutritious meat. But what happens when you eat thousands of pieces of medicine-filled meat over several decades of your lifetime?

Ironically, massive use of antibiotics is causing new diseases, because it promotes the development of new strains of bacteria that can resist many different antibiotics. These new bugs pose a bigger threat to animals and people than the original bacteria! And if you suspect that you're sensitive to yeast, any extra antibiotics in your system will encourage *Candida* to multiply. Public concern about antibiotics and other powerful drugs in meat has prompted growing demand for "free-range" or "range-fed" meat and poultry, as well as organic eggs. Many supermarkets and even take-out chicken joints now carry meat from animals raised on a natural, drug-free diet.

Since yeast's effects can extend way beyond stomach ailments, you may want to know more about it. See the "Sources" section, which lists some helpful books. And for a new remedy for digestive trouble caused by yeast, look to the discussion of yogurt in Week Five of the Hoffman Program.

The Hoffman Pain-Stopper Diet

Now that you're familiar with some of the prime suspects in food-intolerance cases, you're ready to find out which food criminal is responsible for your upset stomach. Unless your food sensitivities are legion, you need about two weeks to identify troublemakers, using my Pain-Stopper Diet. Here's how it works. First, you take all potential offenders out of your diet for a while. Then you see if your digestive troubles improve. Next, you reintroduce prime suspects into your diet one by one. If your symptoms return, you know what to avoid in the future. My method is time-consuming but foolproof. So do try to be patient; don't give up before you've nabbed your personal dietary offenders.

Instead of limiting meals to foods that usually don't provoke allergic reactions or signs of intolerance, some people prefer a complete fast, drinking only water. This need not be harmful, but you shouldn't try it unless you're under a doctor's supervision, and unless you're on vacation, so you can slow down and rest during the day if necessary.

Serious food-allergy investigators used to recommend that you limit your diet for one week to rice, a single meat, like lamb, a single fruit, like pears, and distilled or spring water. But this diet isn't very nutritious, and it is *very* boring. Instead, if you simply rule out all the foods listed first in each of the following groups, you will automatically eliminate foods responsible for digestive problems.

- *Meat:* You *should not* eat preserved or prepared meats like meat loaf, sausages, hot dogs, cured bacon or ham, breaded meats, meat gravies, cold cuts.

You *may* eat fresh, preferably organic meats like lean beef and pork, lamb, turkey, chicken, game.

- *Fish:* You *should not* eat any breaded fish.

You *may* eat any variety of raw or cooked fish and shellfish. (Personally, I would have a terrible time giving up sushi.)

- *Vegetables:* You *should not* eat potatoes, onions, canned and frozen corn, popcorn, tomatoes, mushrooms, cabbage, broccoli, cauliflower, Brussels sprouts, beans and lentils.

You *may* eat all other fresh vegetables, raw or cooked. And you *may* eat tofu, or bean curd.

- *Fruit:* You *should not* eat any citrus fruits, such as oranges or grapefruit, or blended juices, apples or apple juice, grapes, berries or other fruits with a great many seeds, or dried fruits like raisins.

You *may* eat any other fruits, including pears, melon, bananas. But I suggest you eat fruits in moderation: limit yourself to one a day. If you're worried about consuming enough vitamin C, take extra supplements.

- *Cereals:* You *should not* eat bread, noodles, cakes, pasta, pretzels, crackers, bread crumbs or croutons, biscuits, cereals, or anything else likely to contain wheat, corn, rye, oats, or barley. Watch out for hidden grains in foods like popcorn, corn syrup, processed or canned foods.

You *may* eat white, brown, wild, puffed rice or rice cereals, rice cakes, tapioca, millet, hot or cold cereals made from buckwheat (kasha), quinoa, or amaranth. Like quinoa, amaranth is a grain cultivated by the Aztecs that is relatively high in protein. However, it is low in fat, cholesterol, and gluten, which means it is an excellent food if you have food allergies or sensitivities. You *may* also eat pastas made from amaranth, pure Jerusalem artichoke, or buckwheat, rice or soy flour.

- **Cooking Oils:** You *should not* cook with corn, vegetable, cottonseed, or peanut oils.

You *may* use safflower or olive oil, as well as soy, sesame, pumpkin, sunflower, and canola (rapeseed) oil.

- **Dairy Products:** You *should not* drink cow's milk (whole, skim, condensed, or dried), or eat butter, margarine, yogurt, cheese, buttermilk, ice cream, sherbet, so-called nondairy creamers (they may contain casein, a dairy protein), canned or cream soups, cream sauces or gravies, cocoa mixes, pancakes, waffles, puddings, and baking mixes. Check labels on breads and prepared foods to avoid hidden dairy ingredients.

You *may* drink unflavored soy milk—but check the label for added corn oil or sweeteners such as cane juice, barley malt, or rice syrup.

- **Eggs:** You *should not* eat any raw or cooked eggs, or any prepared foods that may contain powdered eggs or egg whites. Among foods to avoid are baked goods, egg noodles, mayonnaise, salad dressings, hollandaise sauce, candies, custards, meringues, and soufflés.

- **Yeast:** You *should not* eat brewer's, baker's or torula yeast, yeast extract, marmite, biscuits, vinegars, alcoholic beverages, ketchup, commercial soy sauce, mushrooms, horseradish, or bouillon cubes unless they are yeast-free. Avoid prepared foods that contain any form of sugar—glucose, sucrose, dextrose, maltose, maltodextrin, fructose, or sweeteners like sorbitol or xylitol (found in gum and soft drinks).

- **Nuts:** You *should not* eat seeds, nuts, and nut butters.

- **Beverages:** You *should not* drink coffee—fresh, instant, or decaffeinated—tea, colas, diet colas, vegetable or fruit juice, alcoholic beverages, tap water, or carbonated water.

You *may* drink herb tea, distilled or spring water. You *may* use tap water for cooking.

- **Seasonings and Additives:** You *should not* use mustard, black or chili pepper, vinegar or bottled salad dressings. You *should not* use chocolate, honey, preservatives, food colorings, or MSG. And you *should not* use regular toothpaste, which contains natural and artificial sweeteners, as well as chemicals and colorings.

You *may* season with salt, white pepper, dried or fresh herbs and spices in moderation. For salad dressings, use olive or sesame oil, combined with pinches of seasonings. To brush your teeth, use baking soda.

You may feel bored on the Hoffman Pain-Stopper Diet, but you need not go hungry. Basically, my diet requires you to stick to fresh, simple foods—nothing canned or prepackaged—so you may have to put in extra time in the kitchen. To keep track of how the limited number of foods you're eating affect you, keep a log during the first week that you follow my Pain-Stopper Diet (see illustrated form for log).

After seven days, 40 percent of patients with food allergies and intolerances feel a marked improvement; their digestive symptoms have disappeared. In fact, by the fifth day, many allergy patients tell me they'd forgotten how it felt to be so well! If you're still feeling any discomfort, perhaps you ate the wrong food by mistake. If that's what happened, start the Pain-Stopper Diet over again the next week.

But perhaps my Pain-Stopper Diet still contains some foods that are problematic for you. To play absolutely safe, try limiting yourself for one week to lamb, peaches, pears, sweet potatoes, millet, and rice, supplemented by an unflavored, hypoallergenic protein powder. If you find that even this minimal diet does not leave you symptom-free, you may have to fast for a minimum of four days. Then, if your symptoms have subsided, you can start reintroducing foods you suspect are problems for you. If you go this route, drink lots of water and be sure to ask a nutrition-oriented M.D. to supervise you.

LINING UP THE SUSPECTS

Once you've found a version of the Hoffman Pain-Stopper Diet that leaves you symptom-free, take another week to start eating possible problem foods again—one food or food group at a time.

- On Monday, add dairy products to your basic diet.
- On Tuesday, if you feel no digestive discomfort, start eating grains that contain gluten—wheat, rye, barley, oats.

HOFFMAN PAIN-STOPPER DIET PROGRESS LOG

	Breakfast	Lunch	Dinner	Snack	Symptoms
DAY # ___ OF DIET Date: _____ Foods eliminated: Problem foods added:					
DAY # ___ OF DIET Date: _____ Foods eliminated: Problem foods added:					
DAY # ___ OF DIET Date: _____ Foods eliminated: Problem foods added:					
DAY # ___ OF DIET Date: _____ Foods eliminated: Problem foods added:					
DAY # ___ OF DIET Date: _____ Foods eliminated: Problem foods added:					
DAY # ___ OF DIET Date: _____ Foods eliminated: Problem foods added:					
DAY # ___ OF DIET Date: _____ Foods eliminated: Problem foods added:					

- On Wednesday, if your stomach is still settled, add gaseous foods: the cabbage family—Brussels sprouts, broccoli, cauliflower—as well as nuts, carbonated water, fruits and other foods containing fructose.
- On Thursday, if you continue to feel fine, you can start eating eggs once more.
- On Friday, you can enjoy potatoes again.
- On Saturday, you may eat anything you like that contains yeast, and you may put vinegar on your salads.
- On Sunday, you can finally have some chocolate.

Any day that you reintroduce a food you've eliminated for a week, eat generous amounts of that food to ensure a noticeable reaction. For example, on Monday, when you're testing milk, drink milk (without adding chocolate, malt, or other flavorings), but also slather butter on your Ry-Crisp, and eat cottage cheese for lunch.

Continue to keep your log! Note very carefully when you add each food and any subsequent digestive trouble you have. Symptoms of intolerance appear fairly quickly:

- Heartburn and dyspepsia usually occur about a half-hour after eating.
- Gas, bloating, and diarrhea begin within 3 to 4 hours, but may develop as late as 18 to 24 hours later.
- Rectal burning or itching may start from 18 to 72 hours after eating.

If you have any symptoms of intolerance, stop eating the foods you added back that day. Or depending on your symptoms, as listed here, and how quickly they set in, check your log to see what foods you reintroduced one to three days ago, and cut those particular foods out. Wait until all your discomfort subsides. You may not be sensitive to every food in the group you resumed eating. But you know that you've spotted a category you should reexamine in more detail. For example, if you had a bad reaction to fruit, try testing only citrus, a group that gives many people digestive trouble.

Once you've nailed the troublemakers in one category, wait until your symptoms clear up, and then test the next group of suspect foods on your list. If you discover that you are sensitive to more than one food, my Pain-Stopper Diet will take you longer than two weeks.

While eliminating and then reintroducing troublesome foods is simple enough, it does require patience, persistence, and careful record-keeping. Try to avoid the common pitfall of stopping before you've finished your dragnet and have a definitive list of your Most Wanted food criminals.

LIVING WITH FOOD INTOLERANCE OR ALLERGY

Once you've fingered the foods that give you trouble, ban them from your diet for a whole month. Sometimes an allergy or sensitivity develops because you have been eating a certain food too often. If this is the case, you may be able to enjoy it once in a while if you rotate your diet, eating only every five days a food you might be sensitive to. Unhappily, this usually doesn't work with lactose or gluten intolerance. In those cases, you have to "just say no": give up milk and wheat products completely.

By the end of your two or more weeks on my Pain-Stopper Diet, you'll have a clear idea of where your dietary pitfalls lie on any menu. You may feel a pang if you have to say goodbye to special favorites. Remember my patient who had to relinquish chocolate, raspberries, whipped cream and even champagne? Certainly she had to give up the good life in gourmet terms. But she soon reported that being rid of stomach pain that struck three times a week was well worth the price. And after all, she could still relish caviar.

Week Five: Eat More

"Those guys eating were like a woman packing a trunk—it's not a question of capacity, but of how much she has to put in."

—Archie Goodwin, Nero Wolfe's assistant,
observes his boss and a dozen
master chefs at a banquet, in
Too Many Cooks, *by Rex Stout*

I'm not about to go on indefinitely asking you to eliminate foods from your diet—and mostly your favorites, at that! Now I want to talk about foods that actually help you avoid digestive trouble. In most cases, you can pack in a trunk-load full of them if you like. Some of these foods are familiar, but others may sound fairly exotic.

Drops and Drops to Drink

As you discovered in Chapter 2, when we took a quick trip down your gastrointestinal tract, digestion requires water—a great deal of it. If you've ever signed up for Weight Watchers, or spent any time flipping through magazine articles on health or beauty, you've heard over and over again that you should drink at least six to eight glasses of water every day. If you have chronic digestive trouble, you may have gotten the same prescription from nutritionists or enlightened gastroenterologists.

Hoary as this advice may be, it works. So do drink those six to eight glasses, even if you have to line them up on the kitchen counter every morning, or keep a bottle of mineral water at work so you can take quick swigs during the day. Some water lovers arrive at their jobs with a gallon jug, and try to finish it before they go home. (For the sake of our environment, make sure you buy returnable glass bottles, rather than plastic ones, which aren't biodegradable. Bottled mineral water is usually safer than tap water, as I'll explain in the next chapter.)

Once you start drinking enough water, some gastric problems, like constipation, clear up quickly. One Iranian researcher actually used water as an ulcer medication. He studied some prisoners with ulcers, presumably while he was imprisoned himself. He had these prisoners drink a great deal of water, and they found that their ulcers healed.

Rewards from Roughage

Today Americans have become extremely conscious of fiber as a cholesterol fighter—so much so that oat-bran muffin makers say they can get any price for their product. But until 1976, the fashionable view of fiber was that you should avoid it. Because fiber is not digested, medical thinking went, it might irritate your gastrointestinal tract. Then British researchers Hugh C. Trowell and Denis P. Burkitt pointed out that Africans have both low cholesterol levels and little incidence of bowel cancer, thanks to a daily diet that's very high in fiber.

The term "dietary fiber," coined by Trowell and Burkitt, refers to a diverse group of foods that work in different ways but synchronize to help you digest. There are two basic groups of fiber, each of which has its own special effects on your body. Soluble fibers, of which modish oat bran is just one example, dissolve in water. They appear to reduce cholesterol levels in your blood, both by speeding cholesterol out of your body and by preventing your small intestine from fully absorbing it.

While soluble fibers work like a whisk, insoluble fibers soak up like a sponge. Insoluble fibers, sometimes called crude fibers, do not dissolve in water. Instead, they sop up water in your intestine. One familiar type of insoluble fiber, wheat bran, can absorb up to three times its weight in water. When insoluble fibers reach your colon, your internal flora can only partly break them down. The result: insoluble fibers act like a natural laxative. You have softer, heavier stools that you can pass effortlessly. And you have them sooner after meals: insoluble fiber speeds up the time it takes fecal matter to pass through your colon.

Eating more insoluble fiber can liberate you from constipation and fend off diverticulosis, irritable bowel syndrome, and hemorrhoids. Burkitt believes that lack of insoluble fiber is the reason diverticulosis is common in Western countries, especially in North America. When you are constipated, you strain to expel your stool. This pressure is a major cause of hemorrhoids, and may also leave pockets in the lining of your colon. This chronic condition is diverticulosis. Once these pockets form, they may easily become inflamed when food particles and bacteria are trapped in them. Then you have an attack of diverticulitis, a serious and painful illness.

Since their pioneering study, both Trowell and Burkitt have speculated that fiber eaters are less prone to colon cancer because fiber speeds the time waste products take to pass through your digestive tract. Hence, any carcinogens you ingest with your food, as well as bodily substances like bile and harmful microbes, which become dangerous if they linger in your gut, are flushed out with your feces.

But the typical American's low-fiber diet allows waste to move sluggishly through your digestive system. Too much fat in your diet increases the amount of bile in your colon. Fiber, however, binds toxic and potentially carcinogenic compounds and carries them swiftly, along with bacteria and other potential irritants, through and out of your colon. Fiber also absorbs and dilutes bile acids, so that you excrete more in a less potent form.

In the past hundred years, sugar, in the diet of the West, has more and more replaced complex carbohydrates, which include fibrous foods. Trowell found that in England, the average daily consumption of cereals, a major source of fiber, fell from 500 grams per person in 1770, to 400 in 1860, to 300 in 1910, to 200 in 1970. Today, most Westerners eat only 5 to 15 grams of fiber each day. Here's just one example that shows how this decline came about: compared to fresh tomatoes, canned tomatoes contain 39 percent less fiber overall.

Most of us need to boost our fiber intake to around 25 to 40 grams a day. Weight Watcher members are familiar with the injunction to eat all the fresh vegetables they want, to quell hunger pangs. Fiber fills you up, and also is chock-full of vitamins and minerals for even more cancer protection. Wheat bran and grains are your best sources of insoluble fiber. Soluble fiber comes from fruit (but *not* juices, so you should eat whole fresh or dried fruit, and preferably the skin as well), legumes, dried peas, beans, and lentils, barley and oats, as well as gums like guar and oat gum. You often eat these sticky fibers without realizing they're in your food. If you've ever cooked hot oatmeal from whole grains, you've seen oat gum: it's the sticky sauce the grains are bathed in after boiling for an hour or so. Another good source of soluble fiber is psyllium, an Oriental seed which comes from plantain. The main ingredient in Metamucil, it's now being marketed in cereal. It's a wonderful alternative if you happen to be allergic to gluten in oat bran, and it lowers cholesterol, too.

Yes, You Can Have Too Much of a Good Thing

If you suddenly switch to a high-fiber diet, you may suffer from gas and bloating, especially if you eat beans. Cookbooks often recommend that you lessen flatulence by soaking the beans overnight, rinsing them, and then adding fresh water to cook them. You will indeed have less gas, but also fewer vitamins from the beans.

A better way to avoid discomfort is to gradually increase your fiber intake, and to eat beans that are less apt to form gas—white beans, chick peas, limas, and lentils. Drink plenty of water as well. Now you need it more than ever, to help fiber move efficiently through your digestive system without irritating it. If you take these steps, gas generally disappears within two to three weeks.

If it doesn't, perhaps your problem is fiber overload. The fact that fiber is so much in vogue right now in cholesterol-conscious America has led to severe cases of fiber overdosing. There have been several reports of patients with large and small intestines stopped up by bezoars, blockages of unprocessed bran that has mixed with bile and salts and turned hard as concrete! One 75-year-old man who had had colon surgery for diverticulitis suddenly started eating muffins heavily laced with oat bran. After only a few days, he began to feel nausea, to vomit frequently. He had abdominal pain and at the same time, no bowel movements. In the hospital, his x-rays showed signs of obstruction in the small intestine. When his surgeons operated, they removed a solid bran bezoar two feet long! Apparently, this man's ability to digest had been slowed by his previous operation. So his sudden switch to a very high-bran muffin habit had completely overwhelmed his small intestine's ability to handle so much fiber.

Of course, this man got into trouble because he was an exceptional fiber consumer. You can certainly eat more fiber without bad effect,

---

HOW TO EAT MORE FIBER

Here are three easy, tasty diets for getting more fiber into your day. You can substitute many interesting ethnic dishes that incorporate fiber: pasta primavera, meatless chili, bean burritos, bean-rice dishes, white or brown rice, moo goo gai pan, pad thai (a Thai noodle specialty), black bean soup, gazpacho, dal (spicy Indian gravy made from legumes), vegetable curry, basmati rice with vegetables, couscous, tabouleh, hummous, and baba-ganoush.

10-GRAM FIBER DIET

	Measure	*Fiber (g)*
BREAKFAST		
Special K	1 cup	—
Milk, 1% fat	¾ cup	—
Orange juice	¾ cup	0.4
White bread, toasted	1 slice	0.6
Egg, soft boiled	1 medium	—
LUNCH		
Tuna sandwich		
Tuna, water-pack	2 oz.	—
Light mayonnaise	1 Tbsp.	—
Celery	½ stalk	0.3
White bread	2 slices	1.0

(continued from opposite page)

Salad		
Lettuce, iceberg	1 cup	0.6
Cucumber	⅛ cup	0.1
Tomato	¼	0.4
French dressing (reduced calorie)	1 Tbsp.	—
Apple juice	¾ cup	0.2
Peach	1	1.4

SNACK		
Grapes	10	0.4

DINNER		
Turkey, light, no skin	4 oz.	—
Mashed potato	¾ cup	2.4
Butter	1 pat	—
Green beans, canned	½ cup	0.9
White roll	1	1.1
Grape juice	1 cup	0
Ice cream	8 oz.	—

SNACK		
Graham crackers	2 pieces	0.5
Milk, 1% fat	1 cup	—

Daily Total for 10-Gram Diet
Calories: 2,020; Fat: 25% of calories;
Protein: 105 g; Calcium: 1,099 mg;
Fiber: 10.3 g.

(continued on page 106)

(continued from page 105)

20-GRAM FIBER DIET

	Measure	*Fiber (g)*
BREAKFAST		
Wheaties	1 cup	3.0
Banana	½ medium	0.9
Milk, 1% fat	¾ cup	—
Orange juice	¾ cup	0.4
Whole wheat toast	1 slice	2.2
LUNCH		
Salad		
Spinach	1 cup	1.4
Carrot, shredded	¼ cup	0.9
Mushrooms	¼ cup	0.3
Italian dressing (reduced calorie)	1 Tbsp.	—
Cheese sandwich		
Wheat bread	2 slices	1.8
Swiss cheese	1.5 oz.	—
Lettuce	1 piece	0.2
SNACK		
Rye crackers	2	2.2
Peanut butter	1 Tbsp.	1.0
Milk, 1% fat	1 cup	—
DINNER		
Stir-Fry		
Chicken, light, no skin	4 oz.	—
Onion	¼ cup	0.6
Broccoli	¼ cup	1.0
Carrots	¼ cup	0.9
Oil	1 Tbsp.	—

(continued from opposite page)

Brown rice	¾ cup	2.5
Pineapple, diced	½ cup	0.9
Yogurt	1 cup	—
Cranberry cocktail	6 oz.	—

SNACK

Popcorn, air-popped, unsalted	2 cups	2.6
Grape juice	¾ cup	0

Daily Total for 20-Gram Diet
Calories: 1,969; Fat: 24% of calories;
Protein: 106 g; Calcium: 1,760 mg;
Fiber: 22.8 g.

30-GRAM FIBER DIET

	Measure	Fiber (g)
BREAKFAST		
Shredded Wheat	1 biscuit	3.0
Milk, 1% fat	¾ cup	—
Bagel	1 plain	1.4
Grapefruit	½	0.7
Orange juice	¾ cup	0.4
LUNCH		
Bean salad		
Lima beans	¼ cup	3.4
Green beans	¼ cup	0.5
Kidney beans	¼ cup	4.6
Oil & vinegar	1 Tbsp	—

(continued on page 108)

(continued from page 107)

Tuna sandwich

Tuna, water-pack	2 oz.	—
Light mayonnaise	1 Tbsp.	—
Celery	½ stalk	0.3
Whole wheat bread	2 slices	4.1
Grape juice	1 cup	—
Peach	1	1.4

SNACK

Carrot	1	2.3
Yogurt	1 cup	—

DINNER

Cod	6 oz.	—
Yogurt topping	1 Tbsp.	—
Corn	½ cup	3.1
Broccoli	½ cup	2.6
French bread	1.5 oz.	1.0
Butter	1 pat	—
Ice milk	¾ cup	—

SNACK

Peanuts, dry roasted	¼ cup	2.9
Cranberry juice cocktail	6 oz.	—

Daily Total for 30-Gram Diet
Calories: 2,126; Fat: 20% of calories;
Protein: 121 g; Calcium: 1,248 mg;
Fiber: 31.7 g.

© 1990, Center for Science in the Public Interest. Reprinted from *Nutrition Action Healthletter,* June 1984 (1501 16th Street, N.W., Washington, D.C. 20036. $19.95 for ten issues.)

provided you don't start eating massive amounts. And alternate your fiber sources: every couple of days, switch from wheat breakfast cereal (full of insoluble fiber) to rice or oats (good for soluble fiber). Eat whole grains, fruits, and vegetables; don't expect sprinkling oat or wheat bran on everything you eat to suffice. And beware of oat-bran muffins: while oat bran itself is certainly good for you, it is no more or less effective than any other soluble fiber. And most oat-bran muffins are cakes in disguise—loaded with calories and oozing fat.

You Never Outgrow Your Need for Calcium

You don't really have to drink milk all your life—although the American Dairy Association would be most happy if you did. You *do* have to make sure you always get plenty of calcium. Milk and dairy products are excellent sources of calcium, but there are others that are less fatty and may be easier for you to digest.

Calcium is a mineral found in the earth, one of twenty-two that are vital to your body's proper functioning. Although calcium is the most plentiful mineral in your body, found mostly in your bones and teeth, you can't manufacture it; you have to obtain it by eating or drinking the right nourishment. Unfortunately, it's actually pretty easy *not* to get enough calcium: under the best of circumstances, your body absorbs only about 15 to 35 percent of the calcium you eat. And you have to be careful about eating certain foods that actively prevent calcium absorption.

Normally, your bones serve as a large reservoir of calcium, releasing it daily into your bloodstream. Besides maintaining strong bones and teeth, calcium is an important nutrient for your colonic cells, and is key to the way your body's cells function. They communicate constantly in chemical code, using calcium channels. When you have enough calcium so that the "calcium connection" is well maintained, cells don't divide needlessly, building up polyps, which are unusual extensions of the lining of your colon into the space through which your food passes. You probably remember hearing a good deal about colorectal polyps when President Reagan was in office. He may not have been eating calcium-rich meals frequently enough: when the calcium level in your food drops, cells can't send messages to each other, and eventually they start dividing when they shouldn't. The results, polyps, aren't cancerous themselves, but they do warn you that there's a precancerous condition in your colon, where abnormally fast cell division is speeding your body in cancer's direction.

Calcium's importance as a cancer preventive is even more evident when you consider that colon cancer is now the second most common cancer in this country, after lung cancer. Calcium seems to keep cell proliferation at a minimum. In your colon, calcium combines with harmful bile acids and fatty acids, so that they pass out of your body without irritating your intestinal lining.

Scientists first began to speculate about calcium's ability to block cancer when they noticed that in Scandinavia, where colon cancer rates are very low, milk consumption is high. Then two researchers, Cedric Garland and his brother Frank, recently carried the calcium connection one step farther. They mapped incidence of intestinal cancer in the United States, and noticed that sunny states, like California and New Mexico, had low rates. Northeastern cities, like Boston, New York, and Washington, where President Reagan, a Californian, happened to be living when doctors found his colorectal polyps, had high colon cancer rates. The Garlands suggested that sunlight made such a crucial difference because the sun's ultraviolet rays help manufacture vitamin D in your body. In turn, vitamin D helps you absorb calcium.

Widening their mapping project to the whole world, the Garlands discovered that "rates of colorectal cancer were higher in places in the world with the least sunlight, such as regions distant from the equator, and in the 'concrete canyons' of large metropolitan areas." The brothers noted that even a row of ten-story buildings, low by some cities' standards, can block sunlight from the street below. Surprisingly, some rural areas, like New Hampshire, Maine, and parts of Canada, also had many cases of intestinal cancer. The Garlands deduced that pollution from industrial areas was blocking country sunlight just as effectively as skyscrapers.

By contrast, sunny places all over the world, "from North Africa to the Caribbean to Central America, had very low rates of colon cancer, vanishing to nearly zero in equatorial Africa." There were few exceptions to this worldwide pattern. But one was milk-loving Scandinavia, where winters are long and dark. Another major exception was Japan, which is at the same latitude as San Francisco and receives about the same amount of sunlight. However, San Francisco's colorectal cancer rates are extremely high, while Japan's are very low.

The Garlands thought the Japanese diet provided a clue explaining this discrepancy. There is one striking way Japanese menus differ from most Western ones: like Scandinavians, Japanese consume enormous amounts of fish, which are generally rich in vitamin D. Japanese are particularly fond of anchovies, sardines, smelts, and other small species that thrive near the ocean's surface and hence are exposed to sunlight, absorbing plenty of vitamin D. Another Japanese favorite, salmon, contains a great deal of vitamin D. And anago, a type of eel that is a choice feature at sushi bars, is the world's richest natural source of vitamin D. The Japanese diet also is low in fat, which can bind calcium, making it harder for your body to absorb it.

HOW TO GET ALL THE CALCIUM YOU NEED
The Garlands believe that a high-fat diet can lead to calcium deficiency, so anyone eating like a normal American may be susceptible. If you live where there's plenty of sunlight, you need less vitamin D in your diet, but if you live up north or in a heavily polluted place, you need *more* calcium and *more* vitamin D to fend off intestinal cancer. I don't recommend spending extra time in the sun nowadays; thanks to ozone depletion, you risk skin cancer from too many ultraviolet rays. It's far

---

CALCIUM-RICH FOODS

There are ways to get all the calcium you need without relying on dairy products. For example, instead of nonfat milk, choose foods that are also high in calcium, such as sunflower seeds and cooked dried beans, or any of the following:

- calcium-fortified soymilk
- broccoli, collard greens, or bokchoy
- almonds
- turnip greens
- kale or mustard greens
- beet greens
- quick-cooking, enriched farina
- enriched cornbread

---

better to eat more fish, along with calcium-rich foods. See the accompanying list for the calcium stars.

• Basically, you should double your calcium intake—especially if you're still drinking any alcohol, coffee, tea, or caffeinated colas. Usually your kidneys conserve calcium, but caffeine and alcohol cause them to excrete much more. That's one reason why a time-honored treatment for a hangover is a large dose of calcium the morning after; you begin to feel much better once you replace the stores you've lost.

• If you're obliged to take certain drugs, including tetracycline, thyroid preparations, or diuretics, you need extra calcium. Antacids containing aluminum are bad enough, but another reason to avoid them is that they decrease calcium absorption.

• Eating a great deal of protein and another mineral, phosphorus, also robs you of calcium. Most Americans, who tend to eat generous quantities of meat and soft drinks, are absorbing two to three times as much protein and three times as much phosphorus as they need.

• Vary your diet, so that you are not relying heavily on other foods that are calcium robbers (discussed next). Their molecules bond very easily to calcium. Then, instead of being absorbed, calcium passes right through your body and is excreted, doing you no lasting good at all.

BEWARE OF CALCIUM THIEVERY

Oddly, some kinds of fiber, which I just finished telling you are so beneficial, are ruthless calcium robbers. Particular villains include bran, believe it or not, as well as coconut, walnuts, pecans, peanuts and peanut butter. Some fibrous foods themselves contain impressive amounts of calcium: rhubarb, beet greens, chard, kale, spinach, and soybeans are good examples. But these foods also contain oxalates, substances that hinder calcium absorption. Fresh rhubarb pie is very hard to resist, so your best strategy is to top it off with some yogurt. If you like spinach salad, drink some milk along with it. Then the oxalates will bind the calcium in the fruit or vegetable, but leave the yogurt or milk's content free for your body to use.

Another good source of fiber, grains, have calcium blockers called phytates in their outer husks. Baker's yeast destroys some phytates, so bread will steal less of your calcium. When you enjoy whole-grain oatmeal or barley or bulgur wheat, used in tabouleh, a Middle Eastern specialty, make sure you also eat calcium-rich foods at other meals.

But if fiber is such a calcium thief, what about Trowell and Burkitt's findings, that colon cancer is so low in Africa? The two British researchers attributed Africans' good health to their fiber-rich diet. Doesn't all that fiber rob them of calcium? How do they defend themselves from colon cancer? Part of the answer is that Africans don't consume bran; they get almost all their fiber from fruits and vegetables. And thanks to their sunny continent, they have high levels of vitamin D to help absorb calcium.

Another factor in Africans' favor is that they may be choosing the right kind of fiber: not all types block your calcium absorption. One variety of soluble fiber, pectin, found in most fruits and vegetables, actually helps you absorb calcium. Especially good pectin sources are apples, kiwis, figs, citrus fruits, broccoli, Brussels sprouts, cucumbers, carrots, cabbage, tomatoes, lima beans, onions, cauliflower, and dark leafy vegetables like watercress, turnip greens, mustard greens. If you cannot tolerate lactose, or prefer your calcium without dairy, eat pectin-rich foods as often as you can.

And since many calcium stealers are very good for you in other ways, still another nutritional strategy is to get your fiber from as many different foods as possible, rather than just sprinkling cereals and salads with bran. If you eat a varied diet, including pectin as well as calcium robbers, your calcium absorption won't drop significantly.

WHAT ABOUT SUPPLEMENTS?

If you must take calcium supplements, because you want to ward off osteoporosis, many doctors recommend calcium carbonate, which contains the most calcium of any available supplement—40 percent. If you take it in the form of Tums, as many people do, it is also inexpensive. But downing large doses of any antacid can do your digestive system more harm than good. And if you have hypochlorhydria, or poor secretion of stomach acid—a common condition in older people —you may not absorb calcium carbonate efficiently because the antacid has neutralized the acid you have left. Proper calcium absorption requires your stomach to be acidic. A better bet is calcium citrate. It is an acidic form of calcium, and your digestive tract absorbs calcium best in an acidic environment. However, calcium citrate is not so acidic that it will upset your stomach.

Many calcium-supplement shoppers were impressed by a 1986 study from the University of Maryland's School of Pharmacy. This study maintained that a simple home test, dropping a calcium tablet in six ounces of ordinary, room-temperature vinegar, could help you judge how well your digestive tract would absorb it. If a calcium tablet is to be absorbed well, three quarters of it, the Maryland study said, should dissolve in the vinegar within a half-hour.

In fact, this vinegar test is useless. The truth is that many less-expensive calcium supplements dissolve faster in vinegar because they are made with poor-quality binders to hold the tablets together. The fact that these supplements fall apart easily doesn't necessarily mean that your gut absorbs them better. This study totally ignores what we know about the physiology of digestion: besides stomach acid, other processes, including the stomach's churning and peristalsis, go to work to help you digest calcium, along with other nutrients.

Finally, before you go supplement-shopping, consider whether you've overlooked a ubiquitous source of calcium—tap water. In some cities, the municipal water supply contains only 26 milligrams of calcium per quart, so you will need to eat calcium-rich foods as well. But in other places where the local water is hard—that is, contains high concentrations of calcium and another mineral, magnesium—its calcium content may be as high as 200 milligrams per quart. In that case, the Garlands point out, you can get up to one third the calcium you need daily just by drinking about two and a half quarts of water. (The calcium content of bottled mineral water usually isn't listed on the label, but is available from the distributor. For reasons I'll explain in the next chapter, bottled mineral water may be a better choice than tap water.) And you *should* drink plenty of water anyway, to make sure that your calcium is well absorbed.

Vegetables and Herbs That Heal

Guess which fruit or vegetable is Americans' number-one source of nutrients. Perhaps you're pondering the apple or the carrot. The correct answer is the tomato—technically a fruit but, gastronomically speaking, a vegetable. Despite its popularity, however, the tomato, according to a study from the University of California, Davis, is only sixteenth in nutritional value among available crops. Of course, the tomato has its virtues: as I've just noted, it's an excellent source of pectin and therefore helps you absorb calcium. But if you want to eat meals that are as nutritionally sound as possible, you'd be better off if you picked any of the vegetables that outrank the tomato. These include, in descending order, broccoli, spinach, Brussels sprouts, lima beans, peas, asparagus, artichokes, cauliflower, sweet potatoes, carrots, sweet corn, potatoes, and cabbage. Many of these, thanks to their high fiber and/or calcium content, will also help you avoid the very worst digestive problem, colon cancer.

SALADS FROM THE SEA

Besides common vegetables that you may be overlooking, there are some unusual ones that you may never have tasted. They don't appear on the Davis researchers' list, but they certainly have extraordinary nutritional and digestive value. If you like sushi, you've probably sampled one of them: seaweed. The papery black wrapping on sushi rolls is dry nori, a red seaweed.

Seaweeds are marine algae, simple photosynthesizing plants that often lack the leaves, stems, and roots that you're used to seeing in land plants. But sea vegetables are just as diverse. There are over 20,000 different varieties, in four main groups—red, green, brown, and blue-green algae. Sea vegetables are the world's most common food source—and the most underused, except among the Japanese, who eat many kinds of seaweed dishes. Recently, they have won some new American enthusiasts among adherents of the macrobiotic diet.

In truth, you ingest seaweeds often without realizing it. Colloids, a form of fiber that gives brown sea plants their rigidity and strength, are used widely as emulsifiers, thickeners, and stabilizers. They make sherbets, ice cream, chocolate milk, salad dressings, and toothpaste smooth; they render wines clear and beers foamy.

All sea vegetables and mosses are excellent sources of soluble fiber, as well as veritable treasure troves of nutrients. One group alone, brown sea plants—known as kelp—contains ten vitamins, seventeen amino acids, and twenty minerals. You can buy seaweed in health-food stores, which often also offer cooking advice. Most of the varieties you can buy in this country—arame, dulse, hiziki, kombu, nori, wakame—are excellent sources of calcium. Hiziki supplies fourteen times the amount in one glass of milk. Dulse, common in Nova Scotia and Maine, is also the best non-animal source of iron. Kombu, a type of kelp, also is a good kidney and colon cleanser; when cooked with beans, it enhances flavor and helps neutralize the gas they're apt to produce in your digestive tract. Another variety of seaweed, agar, is

If so many vegetables are good for me, should I become a vegetarian?

Well, Plato, Pythagoras, Plutarch, Leonardo da Vinci, Leo Tolstoy, George Bernard Shaw, Albert Einstein, Albert Schweitzer, and even Madonna and Greg Louganis would probably chorus, "By all means!" If you become a vegetarian, you have to be careful to get enough protein from sources like beans. But numerous scientific studies have credited a vegetarian diet with relieving and minimizing the risk of many modern gastrointestinal problems, including constipation, appendicitis, irritable bowel syndrome, gallstones, hemorrhoids, and even colon cancer.

At present I am a vegetarian about 90 percent of the time, and I can attest to the diet's general contribution to good health. Here's one small example of its beneficial effects: some of my patients suffer from anal pruritus, or irritation of the skin around the anus that causes raw, red cracking and itching that can keep you awake at night. Whenever I have been able to persuade such patients to become reasonably conscientious vegetarians, all signs of pruritus cleared up.

What if I don't eat at all? Will fasting help my digestive troubles clear up?

Yes indeed—periodic fasts for 24 hours or so give your digestive tract a chance to rest from its laborious, nonstop task of absorbing nutrients from one meal after another. Instead, your gut can devote itself to self-regeneration and forcing toxins out of your body.

Be sure to fast over a weekend so that you can rest if necessary. You don't have to avoid aerobic exercise completely, but don't try to test your limits while you're fasting; exercise a little less vigorously. At all times, drink plenty of water—or half-strength juices or vegetable broth. If you have health problems, or have never fasted before, you need a doctor's supervision.

full of fiber, a great remedy for constipation. Both nori and agar also bond with cholesterol and carcinogens, respectively, to carry them out of your body.

Like other elements of the Japanese diet, sea vegetables are high in sodium. However, thorough rinsing can remove most of the salt, and in any case, the sodium may be offset by the plants' high potassium content. In seaweed, the ratio of sodium to potassium is 3 to 1, close to your body's 5 to 1 ratio, and very different from the 10,000 to 1 ratio of table salt.

HOW TO CONQUER VAMPIRES . . . AND CANCER

Recent research has indicated that cruciferous vegetables—members of the cabbage and collard families—help you fend off gastric cancer. Now there are additional findings that another set of vegetables that you might expect to upset your stomach are good cancer fighters. I'm talking about allium vegetables—garlic, onions, leeks, chives, scallions.

One member of this family, garlic, has been a digestive remedy since ancient times. It boosts your immune system and contains a natural antibiotic: raw garlic is more powerful than penicillin or tetracycline. Garlic has been used to combat a long list of bacterial illnesses, including digestive diseases like diarrhea and dysentery. In ancient Rome, Pliny prescribed garlic for gastrointestinal disorders, among them ulcers and hemorrhoids.

Then in 1989, a collaborative study by the National Cancer Institute and Chinese scientists found that garlic, onions, and other allium vegetables provide protection against gastric cancer. This research discovered that Chinese who were free of stomach cancer consumed in an average year at least twenty-five pounds and up to more than fifty pounds of allium vegetables. This isn't an extraordinary amount if you agree with Nora Ephron, who noted in her novel *Heartburn* that "you can't really cook without onions." And some cooks would say the same about garlic.

The scientists involved in the Chinese-American study pointed out that their findings hold true elsewhere: for instance, onion lovers in Greece and Japan also succumb to gastric cancer less frequently. In the United States, around Vidalia, Georgia, where farmers grow distinctively sweet Vidalia onions, available only in late spring and early summer, the rate of stomach cancer among whites is about one-third the national level and one-half the state level. And in a northern Chinese province with the country's lowest rate of gastric cancer, garlic is a major crop. Chinese scientists themselves have noted that garlic and onions can reduce the risk of stomach cancer by as much as 60 percent.

One way that these two vegetables may combat cancer is by boosting your immune system. Chewing on raw garlic will ruin your kisses, but the Japanese extract, Kyolic, leaves no traces on your breath.

"BITTERS, PLEASE"

Once I arrived at the airport with a bad stomachache. My wife had packed dinner for me, but the thought of eating a home-cooked meal —much less airline food—was unthinkable. Not only was I in pain, but I had a long, difficult business trip ahead of me, and I knew I ought to eat if I expected to have the energy I was going to need.

Instead of searching for a counter that sold antacids, I went to a bar. There I asked the barman for mineral water, mixed with an herbal liquor known as bitters. After a couple of glasses, my stomachache had disappeared, and I had a hearty appetite.

The secret cure is the ingredients in the liquor I asked for—bitter herbs, mainly gentian root, probably combined with artichoke leaves, dandelion, yarrow flowers, angelica root, quassia, Peruvian bark (the source of quinine), and bitter orange peel. Fennel and anise seeds add flavor and relief from gas. In Europe, bitters are considered a good after-dinner digestive. Americans are less familiar with bitters and bitter herbs, although Jews refer to bitter herbs at Passover meals, commemorating the bitter experiences of the Hebrews as slaves in Egypt.

Today, bitters are usually considered a remedy for hangover— which is probably why the barman at the airport thought I wanted them! The point is, they soothe the stomach upset that frequently accompanies hangover. They work for both kinds of problems because they flush out toxins by stimulating liver functioning, reducing risk of gallstones at the same time. Besides promoting bile secretion—important for digestion in your small intestine—bitters give you an appetite by stimulating your salivary glands and pepsin secretion in your stomach.

Like garlic, bitter herbs have antibiotic properties. We don't eat many bitter foods—grapefruit, hops, coffee, chocolate and certain greens, including mustard, collard, kale, kohlrabi, green-leaf lettuce, watercress, and artichokes. But like bitter herbs, some bitter foods have digestive benefits. Coffee's bitter properties may explain in part why it often relieves constipation. And currently, the U.S. Department of Agriculture is investigating the ability of bitter compounds in citrus fruit to prevent stomach tumors.

MORE DIGESTION PROTECTION FROM GEORGIA

The morning after a particularly rich dinner, my wife, who is sensitive to fats, often asks me to make her some kudzu (known as kuzu in the macrobiotics community) and umeboshi, or salt plum. First I find some kudzu powder, the starchlike extract of kudzu root, which looks and tastes like milk of magnesia and is just as good for settling and soothing your stomach. Adding some water, a few drops of soy sauce, and a pinch of ginger to the kudzu powder, I bring the mixture to a boil, stirring it into a smooth cream. Then I add a salt plum, which Japanese consider *the* best alkaline food. Soon after she downs my concoction, my wife invariably reports that her acid indigestion is completely gone.

When you've been in gastric pain, most likely you have not reached for kudzu. If you live in or have visited the South, you know that most Southerners consider kudzu a pest and a bad joke, the alien green vine that has invaded their home as memorably as General Sherman. Introduced from Japan because it restores nutrients to soil, kudzu has taken over the American South, where it finds favorable weather and no natural enemies. In Georgia, locals warn you, semiseriously, to close your windows at night to keep kudzu out of your house.

But as the ancient Japanese knew, kudzu can be used in cooking as a thickener like cornstarch or arrowroot flour. Kudzu also has medicinal properties that are particularly effective against gastrointestinal difficulties. It contains a good deal of mucilage, so that when it is made into cream, it coats your stomach. Combined with a salt plum, it is an excellent antidote for acid stomach, gastric pain, or simple overeating. Umeboshi, a wonderful preservative, has antimicrobial properties besides adding alkalinity. These properties go to work in your gastrointestinal tract to eliminate infectious invaders.

There are other effective kudzu-based medicinal preparations and recipes you can sample in *The Book of Kudzu: A Culinary and Healing Guide,* by William Shurtleff and Akiko Aoyagi (published by the Avery

---

Publishing Group, Inc., Wayne, New Jersey, and available in paper-back from The Soyfoods Center, P.O. Box 234, Lafayette, California 94549).

Fermenting a Solution

Sometimes you have digestive trouble because there's a shortage of essential bacteria in your gut. For instance, one of my patients, a man who had had to take massive amounts of antibiotics, was stricken, not surprisingly, with very bad diarrhea and stomach upset. His medication had killed off the microbes that were troubling him—as well as nearly all his colonic bacteria. To begin to restore them, I gave him acidophilus supplements. On his own, he also obtained from Germany capsules of *E. coli,* another bacterium essential to normal colon balance. In Germany, *E. coli* supplements are the mainstay of treatments for digestion gone awry. Lamentably, they are not yet available over here.

A MIRACLE YOU CAN WHIP UP YOURSELF

But other useful bacteria are easy to get—because they're in fermented foods. All over the world, fermented foods have been important parts of various people's diets. One very familiar example is yogurt. Besides being an excellent, low-fat source of calcium, yogurt contains live culture called lactobacilli, which are just about the most available beneficial bacteria.

Yogurt has even been dubbed the "elixir of life" because lactobacilli produce a number of natural antibiotics and can ease diarrhea and gastric pain. They also relieve anal pruritus, intense anal itching and irritation that is often aggravated by a highly alkaline stool—a sure sign that you are deficient in lactobacilli. And they aid digestion for some who cannot tolerate other dairy products.

But some commercial brands of yogurt contain more live culture than others, and frozen yogurt doesn't have any left at all. The best way to ensure that you consume adequate amounts of lactobacilli is to use commercial yogurt as a "starter" for your own homemade variety. This is quite easy—see the accompanying recipe—and the resulting yogurt actually tastes better because it is free of preservatives and artificial flavorings.

HOW TO MAKE YOUR OWN YOGURT

Why bother when it's in every supermarket? Because not all commercial yogurt contains enough healthful lactobacilli to do your digestion good. To make sure you flourish from eating yogurt, the best thing to do is to rely on your own homemade kind. Plus, it usually tastes fresher! If you prefer a high-tech approach, you can buy a yogurt maker from most health-food or gourmet-cookware stores and follow the accompanying directions. You simply put your ingredients in a yogurt maker, plug it in, turn it on, and set the heat at the proper temperature and the right length of time to make your yogurt. Or you can use the following recipe which requires no special equipment at all, except perhaps a cooking thermometer.

You'll need ½ gallon of low-fat milk (I use instant powdered milk), a can of evaporated milk, and a tablespoon of commercial low-fat yogurt (the starter). Plain yogurt from a health-food store is best.

Mix the powdered milk in a large enamel pot. Stir in the evaporated milk, using a wooden spoon. Then *slowly* bring the mixture to a boil, stirring periodically so that the milk doesn't burn or stick to the bottom of the pot. When the milk starts to boil, bubbling to the top of the pot, remove it from the heat and let it cool.

You may add your "starter" when you can insert your finger into the hot milk and count to ten slowly. This method really does work, but if you prefer, you can use a cooking thermometer to find out when the milk has reached the ideal temperature of 105 to 115 degrees Fahrenheit. When the milk is too cool (under 105 degrees), the culture won't work. If you've let the milk cool down too much, reheat it. However, the milk must not be scalding (over 120 degrees), or the living culture, lactobacilli, that makes milk into yogurt will die, and your milk will stay liquid. Generally, slightly cooler milk yields sweeter yogurt; hotter milk makes it tarter.

To add the starter, place it in a cup and fill up the cup with hot milk. Mix the cup's contents with a wooden spoon until they're homogeneous. Pour the mixture into the pot of milk and

(continued on page 122)

(continued from page 121)

stir in one direction only, until everything is thoroughly mixed—about half a minute.

Place five or six layers of paper toweling over the top of the pot, to absorb water as the milk cools and to make your yogurt denser. Then place the pot's lid over the toweling. If you have a gas stove with a pilot light, let the pot stand there overnight. If your stove is electric and has no pilot light, you'll get the same results if you wrap the pot in an old woolen blanket and leave it in a warm place overnight. You can even let it stand on a hot plate, set to a very low heat. In the morning, you should have a fine potful of thick yogurt, ready to add to your breakfast fruit or cereal.

FOODS YOU DON'T HAVE TO DIGEST

Another advantage of fermented foods is that the process of fermentation predigests the particular food for you: by the time you eat it, the fermenting agent has already broken down starch blockers or oligosaccharides, so you benefit fully from the food's nutrients. Fermented foods are also rich in enzymes that help you digest. Normally, your body manufactures enzymes, but if you are ill or aging, you may lose your ability to do so. Then fermented foods are especially helpful.

One such predigested drink, rich in enzymes and lactobacilli, is

HOW TO DRINK YOGURT

Lassi, a yogurt drink popular in India and Afghanistan, is easy to make, full of calcium and lactobacilli to help settle and heal your intestinal tract. In a blender, combine 1½ cups plain low-fat or nonfat yogurt with about ten ice cubes. For different flavors you can add a dozen mint or coriander leaves, ginger, saffron, diced cucumber, or if you like it hot, black pepper or chilis.

"rejuvelac," which you can make yourself from soaking hulled seeds, of a variety of grains, in fresh spring water. Rejuvelac is full of vitamins and a good intestinal cleanser, but its smell of fermenting grain can take over your entire house! I prefer a couple of other predigested, fermented foods, including miso.

While the main nutrient in rejuvelac is grain protein, miso offers soy protein in the form of fermented soybean paste. Like kudzu, miso is a staple in the Japanese diet that macrobiotics adherents have popularized in this country. Made from soybeans, some grains (usually rice or barley), salt and water, and fermented by *Aspergillus oryzae* culture (a mold related to penicillin), miso comes in six basic types that comprise about thirty distinct varieties, mostly savory, some sweet, all delicious.

Fresh miso, which has the consistency of soft peanut butter and ranges in color from dark brown to red, yellow, beige, and creamy white, smells quite like freshly ground coffee. Indeed, most Japanese start their day with a bracing, nutritious cup of miso soup, a familiar hors d'oeuvre to Western devotees of Japanese restaurants. All miso is fermented by adding olive-green koji "starter," or dried spores of aspergillus mold, which functions like sourdough culture in sourdough bread, or like various other molds in mold-ripened cheeses such as Camembert or gorgonzola. Darker, traditional misos are higher in protein and salt, and are made with twice as many soybeans as grain. They are aged in huge wooden vats for at least a year and a half. Mellower misos are lighter in color, and ferment for one to two months. Besides soups, miso makes excellent sauces, dips, and salad dressings. Like yogurt, miso contains lactobacilli and enzymes that aid digestion and fight harmful microbes and contaminants.

Once an exotic specialty found only in Japanese markets, miso is now a staple in most health-food stores. For more about miso, as well as many recipes, consult *The Book of Miso*, also by William Shurtleff and Akiko Aoyagi (Berkeley, California: Ten Speed Press. Available in paperback from Soyfoods Center, P.O. Box 234, Lafayette, California 94549).

Finally, don't forget my own personal favorite: sauerkraut, a familiar fermented dish made from cabbage. If you find that eating cabbage usually gives you gas, try sauerkraut. Like other fermented foods, it actually helps you digest and is very nourishing.

Week Six:
Be Your Own
Digestive Expert

"Indigestion is the forerunner of half the diseases we are liable to."

—*from* An Easy Way to Prolong Life by a
Little Attention to What We Eat and Drink,
by a Medical Gentleman, 1775

If you have been following the Hoffman Program and still have persistent digestive symptoms—chronic pain, perhaps, or loose bowel movements for weeks—you need to see your doctor. But there are clues you can trace to form a pretty clear picture of what's wrong with you. Then you'll have the advantage of knowing what questions to ask your doctor and what kinds of new treatments to consider.

Before you make an appointment, however, you need to find a doctor who is a digestive detective—a nutritionally oriented physician. Conventional gastroenterologists certainly do know exactly how to handle a symptom like blood in your stool. But if your symptoms are more subtle, they may dismiss your concern, or tell you that you're reading too much into your discomfort. (See the "Sources" section for the names of organizations that can put you in touch with sympathetic doctors.)

What Happens in Your Gut to Make You Ill

Whenever you have a digestive disorder, you also have malabsorption in some degree. Malabsorption can be at the root of food allergies, bowel trouble (especially diarrhea), and losing weight for no apparent reason. When you have malabsorption, your gastrointestinal tract cannot break down and absorb nutrients properly. As a result, you may eat a great deal and still have trouble gaining weight, or despite a good diet and plenty of rest, you may feel weak, run-down, and susceptible to colds and flu.

There are several different kinds of malabsorption. It can happen because food passes through your gut much too quickly to be digested properly. When you suffer from diarrhea, you have a classic case of this type of malabsorption. Because malabsorption accompanies diarrhea, anyone who suffers chronic diarrhea for too long will become undernourished.

A second kind of malabsorption occurs if the wall of your large intestine becomes inflamed. This is a major reason why food allergy can trigger malabsorption. For instance, celiac sprue, an extreme form of gluten intolerance, can do so much damage to your intestine's walls that the disease also ranks as an extreme form of this particular type of malabsorption. A *Candida* infection can have a similar effect. Since food allergies and malabsorption often go hand in hand, eliminating problem foods can help some allergic conditions, like childhood asthma and eczema.

You may have a third kind of malabsorption because you lack one of the crucial constituents that make digestion possible. For example, perhaps your liver isn't producing enough bile. You need bile to emulsify fats, and if liver disease has diminished your bile supply, you will not be able to digest fats or fat-soluble vitamins.

Similarly, malabsorption may occur because you have little or no acid in your stomach, or because secretion of your pancreatic enzymes has tapered off as well. Both stomach acid and pancreatic enzymes play major roles in breaking down food in your stomach and small intestine, so that you can then absorb nutrients into your bloodstream and lymphatics. Here's how stomach acid and enzymes *should* work together: first, your stomach acid breaks down your meal into chyme. Then your stomach releases chyme in small spurts into the upper portion of your small intestine, or duodenum. If chyme is

---

sufficiently acid as it enters your duodenum, it stimulates release of pancreatic enzymes.

If your stomach is not sufficiently acidic, your enzyme secretion may in turn dwindle, and the proteins, carbohydrates, and fats you've eaten won't break down enough to provide you with nourishment. But enzyme secretion can slow for other reasons besides lack of stomach acid: as you age, enzyme secretion may diminish, and it can be adversely affected by other factors, including stress, inherited tendencies, and excessive alcohol.

Enzyme production also operates on the principle of "Use it or lose it." A case in point is lactase, the enzyme that enables you to digest lactose. Lactase production tapers off in older people because, in the past, most adults in most cultures did not drink milk. Lactase, then, is useful to babies but not to grown-ups, and so it may gradually peter out as your body ages and you drink milk much less often. There are racial variations, but generally speaking, production of lactase, weakens as you grow older. If this happens to you as you age, you develop lactose intolerance, which qualifies as a type of malabsorption.

Similarly, if you rarely eat fatty foods, you may become deficient in lipase, an enzyme that digests fats. And the longer you go without enough stomach acid to prompt enzyme secretion, the more the delicate interplay and timing of enzyme secretion may be hampered. In any of these instances, when enzyme secretion tapers off, malabsorption may follow.

Although malabsorption is an internal condition, there are obvious signs of it that you can spot yourself. Frequent gas and bloating are among the more obvious. If you suspect that you're being debilitated by malabsorption, you will be able to confirm your suspicion by closely observing your own body, as well as your way of life.

Looking Over Your Life

Various factors, some related to the kind of medical care you may have gotten in the past, can mean that you're at risk for hypochlorhydria (low stomach acid) or, much more rarely, achlorhydria (none at all), and consequently malabsorption.

• *Your Age:* Hydrochloric acid tends to decrease with age, and mild to severe hypochlorhydria is almost universal among people over 65. Your digestive system is an amazing mechanism: it produces all the energy your body needs to function. Since it takes a great deal of energy to produce so much energy, your digestion, just like your body's other energy-producing systems, degenerates over time. When I was 18, I could wolf down two medium-sized pepperoni pizzas on Saturday night at my favorite college restaurant—with great relish and no queasiness on Sunday morning. Now that I'm twice that age, my stomach would balk at that same pizza meal.

• **Your Family Tree:** If you don't know your family's medical history very well, find out whether your grandparents, parents, uncles, aunts, and cousins also have or have had digestive trouble. Perhaps your current intestinal discomfort is an early warning of a serious gastrointestinal illness that runs in your family. Colon cancer, colitis, and food allergies can pass from generation to generation. And while some of us are born with "cast-iron" stomachs, others are colicky and oversensitive from babyhood.

Perhaps you've caught digestive trouble from a relative: there's new evidence that ulcers may be infectious, caused by *Campylobacter* bacteria. (It's just been renamed *Helicobacter*, but still goes by its old name.) Ulcers and other gastric problems can be exacerbated by stress, so if your family tends to react to stress with gastric upset, you may have picked up the habit of reacting this way, too. An Australian study of the psychosocial causes of ulcers noted that "peptic ulcers run in families" for other reasons besides infectious bacteria: "Any cause of prolonged psychological arousal can be associated with high acid secretion and even gastric erosions and bleeding."

Some inherited troubles that seem unrelated to digestion may contribute nonetheless to gastric disturbance. If your relatives tend to have any sort of allergies, you may be susceptible to food sensitivities. Asthma—perhaps because it affects your mucous membranes, which line your lungs as well as your intestines—is also linked to irritable bowel syndrome (IBS). One woman I treated suffered from asthma, as did her mother. While none of my patient's children had asthma, two had IBS. Asthma means a tendency to have spasms in the smooth muscle lining the lungs, and this tendency seems to affect other involuntary muscles, such as those in the colon or the heart. This is the reason why people with a type of heart murmur called mitral valve prolapse—basically an anatomical variation which predisposes you to palpitations—are also susceptible to irritable bowel syndrome or asthma.

I wasn't very surprised that my asthma patient also suffered from arthritis. Poor digestion can bring on "leaky gut syndrome": your digestive tract, which should absorb only nutrients, becomes permeable to many foreign substances as well. Once they enter your circulatory system, they can trigger allergic reactions, including arthritis and asthma.

• **Your Community:** If you and most of your family, your roommates, your fellow workers, or even your neighbors are having repeated bouts of diarrhea, vomiting, or stomach upset, all of you may have shared contaminated food or water. There are about 300 types of foodborne diseases, and many are dangerous to people. Bacteria or viruses can infect meat and poultry, eggs, dairy products, raw fish, and shellfish. One strain, *Salmonella*, taints from 5 to 30 percent of the 5.5 billion broiler chickens raised annually in the United States.

When your stomach acid is already low, you may be especially susceptible to these bugs; an acid gut can resist infection better. In fact, the U.S. Department of Agriculture has tried sweetening the drinking water of broiler chickens with lactose, or milk sugar. This experiment dramatically increased chickens' ability to ward off *Salmonella* infection because lactose made their gut more acidic. Alas, this simple measure does not work for humans!

Sayonara, Sushi?

It grieves me greatly to report that, occasionally, people have been infected with parasites after eating one of my all-time favorite dishes, sushi. Doctors often mistake parasitic infestation for other gastrointestinal illnesses, including colitis, Crohn's disease, irritable bowel syndrome, gallbladder disease, pancreatic problems, ulcers, or even appendicitis. One 24-year-old man who had severe pain in his lower abdomen required exploratory surgery. His surgeon, who was prepared to do a routine appendectomy, was puzzled because his patient's appendix looked quite normal. He glanced a few inches higher, and found that a section of the patient's bowel was very inflamed. The surgeon removed the infected portion, and closed the patient's incision. Only then did the doctor spot a pinkish-red worm about two inches long slinking across the surgical drapes. It turned out to be a nematode parasite common in fish-eating birds.

When the young man came to, his doctors asked about his diet.

Yes indeed, their patient enjoyed sushi or sashimi at least once a month, usually in Japanese restaurants. But the day before his severe abdominal pain had brought him to the hospital, he had eaten home-made sushi at a friend's house.

This need never happen to you if, unlike this patient, you enjoy your sushi only in reputable Japanese restaurants. Both here and in Japan, the great majority of worm infestations from raw fish have resulted from sushi prepared at home. Freshwater fish, or fish like salmon that may be caught in salt water but spend part of their lives in fresh water, may be host to quite a range of parasites that make people sick, including roundworms and flukes. The only risky saltwater fish are mackerel and members of the cod family, including whiting, haddock, and rockfish. Japanese restaurant owners and chefs are specially trained to spot parasite-free fish and to handle it so that it reaches your plate still clean.

As for fish you catch or buy to cook at home, if you have any doubts about its safety, you can freeze it for at least five days at − 4 degrees Fahrenheit (− 20 degrees centigrade). According to the Centers for Disease Control, this temperature kills all parasites tested to date.

Not a Clean Drop to Drink

While you may be safe from parasites in raw fish as long as you eat out, contaminated water is a much more ubiquitous hazard. Americans are so worried about the safety of their drinking water that sales of bottled water and purifying devices have soared 68 percent in the past five years. In 1988 alone, we spent $2 billion on bottled water and $265 million more for purification equipment and services.

And we do have real reason for concern: the National Wildlife Federation documented recently that because the Environmental Protection Agency has failed to enforce the federal law designed to protect public water supplies, public water systems across the country have become polluted. Some 37 million citizens are affected. Thousands of municipalities have discovered unexpectedly high levels of coliform bacteria in their water. Since these bacteria are common in human stool, they are a clear sign that sewage has seeped into reservoirs. Disease-causing bacteria, viruses, parasites, PCBs, pesticides, inorganic compounds like lead, mercury, and arsenic, and even radioactive substances have found their way into ordinary tap water. As a result, a single drink of contaminated water can bring on rapid, debilitating illness, involving at the very least diarrhea and intestinal pain.

Giardia *Alert!*

One of the most frequent causes of waterborne disease in this country is the protozoan *Giardia lamblia,* a microscopic parasite that thrives harmlessly in the intestines of wild animals, especially beavers. As *Giardia* passes out of an animal in its feces, the protozoan forms a protective cyst around itself and remains dormant until it finds another host. Just by defecating, a single beaver can expel *one billion Giardia* cysts per day into a lake or stream.

If the water is cold, this hardy protozoan can survive for at least two months—long enough to find its way into your tap water, especially if you live in a mountainous rural area where your water supply is treated with only standard levels of chlorine. So it's quite possible that a single animal can contaminate an entire municipal water supply. *Giardia* infections have struck residents of Aspen, Colorado, in 1966, northeastern Pennsylvania in 1984, and Missoula, Montana, in 1986.

Besides passing from animal to human, *Giardia* can pass from person to person through sexual contact, contaminated food, or feces. Careless diaper-changing, poor kitchen hygiene, and unsupervised play have caused outbreaks in day-care centers; in some centers, more than half the children have come down with giardiasis. Nationwide, as many as 30 percent of day-care workers may be infected. There have also been outbreaks in mental institutions where hygiene was less than adequate.

In fact, giardiasis is now a national epidemic, affecting from 4 to nearly 8 percent of Americans. Sometimes you have no symptoms— from 7 to 10 percent of the population may be asymptomatic— although you may be able to spread *Giardia* to others. Sometimes giardiasis announces itself in the form of severe symptoms like watery diarrhea and sharp abdominal pain. But it can pass into a chronic form with less acute symptoms that may include fatigue, malaise, mild bloating and gas, and perhaps intermittent diarrhea that you or your doctor can easily mistake for irritable bowel syndrome. In one recent study, nearly one half of patients thought to have irritable bowel syndrome turned out to have giardiasis.

If *Giardia* is spotted, it can be filtered out of municipal water before chlorination, and giardiasis can be treated with drugs and some natural remedies. But if *Giardia* infestation goes undetected for some time, moderate to marked malabsorption and weight loss may ensue. Enzyme secretion may slow, and you can develop lactose intolerance: you may find that eating dairy products or drinking milk makes your giardiasis symptoms worse.

Like other parasites, *Giardia* also can worsen food allergies. *Giardia*'s irritating presence in your gut increases the permeability of your intestinal walls, allowing allergenic food substances to cross into your bloodstream. So if you have any symptoms that suggest a food allergy or intolerance, be sure to ask your doctor for tests to detect parasites, especially *Giardia*. And if you're planning to travel, you'll have to keep a sharp lookout for *Giardia* and other parasites. In the next section, I describe some precautions for travelers.

Your Vacations

If you have spent time recently in Asia, Africa, or Latin America, you may be suffering from "Montezuma's revenge," or traveler's diarrhea. By far the most common health problem associated with travel, hitting up to half of visitors to underdeveloped countries, this type of diarrhea usually follows consumption of food or beverages contaminated by an unfriendly strain of the intestinal bacteria *E. coli* that produces an intestinal toxin. Traveler's diarrhea is particularly common in countries where drinking water and water used to grow and wash food are either tainted with sewage or poorly purified. But nowadays, this scourge also can strike you in industrialized nations—even the United States!—where raw food and tap water are usually considered safe.

While you are away from home, your best bet—especially if you are susceptible to gastric upset—is several ounces of prevention. Eat only well-cooked food or fresh fruits and vegetables with thick skins that you can peel off yourself. Drink only commercially bottled and sealed beverages or water that you are certain has been boiled for at least three minutes. Beer, wine, liquor, and carbonated beverages are fine, but don't add ice. Use bottled water to brush your teeth; don't rely on hot tap water. And ask for bubbly bottled water; in some countries, unscrupulous restaurateurs refill plain mineral-water bottles with tap water, and serve it again!

Traveler's diarrhea usually clears up once you take precautions or return home. Doctors used to recommend that travelers bound for the tropics take antibiotics as a prophylactic, but because these powerful drugs upset your intestinal balance, they actually leave you more prone to infection. On the other hand, one popular nostrum for diarrhea, Pepto-Bismol, contains bismuth, which can help clear up traveler's diarrhea and also may serve you well as a prophylactic. An effective strategy against traveler's diarrhea is to take two Pepto-Bismol tablets four times a day. This regimen will turn your stool black—nothing to worry about—but it will *not* rob you of stomach acid, your best defense against infection. Another effective prophylactic is yogurt capsules: lactobacilli can compete with invaders.

Traveling Companions You Don't Need

A more dangerous and elusive threat than traveler's diarrhea is parasitic infection. Thanks to the *Giardia* epidemic, "Montezuma's revenge" now has an American cousin, "backpacker's lament." Hikers and campers gravitate toward upstate New York, the Great Lakes region, the Pacific Northwest, and Colorado—places where *Giardia* is all too common in limpid mountain lakes and streams. One vacationing Vermonter had managed to avoid *Giardia* at home, even though she lived near a beaver pond, but picked it up from a fountain on the Cape Cod seashore when she ignored a sign that read, "Don't drink the water." No matter how pure the local water looks, boil it before you drink it or cook with it—or take a lightweight camper's water filtering system with you. Don't use iodine tablets to cleanse your drinking water; it's not good for you if you have a potential thyroid problem, and it may not kill off rugged *Giardia* cysts.

Besides being a pest in the United States, *Giardia* is now a problem all over the world, affecting at least 10 percent of the population in some countries. In Leningrad, until recently, neither tourists nor natives could drink tap water, which had been infested with *Giardia*. Other parasites, especially amoebas, are even more prevalent worldwide. In some Third World countries, up to half the inhabitants are infected with amoebas, roundworms, and other parasites.

You may take home *Giardia* and other unwelcome fellow travelers in your intestines by eating or drinking contaminated food or water, or by swimming in infested lakes or rivers. Salt water is generally safe, although after heavy rains the bacterial count at municipal beaches both in the United States and abroad can be high enough to rule out swimming, thanks to runoff from overburdened sewers. Or you may pick up unwanted visitors simply by walking barefoot outdoors: some parasites can enter your body through your feet.

Parasitic infection can be very treacherous. Sometimes you immediately come down with severe dysentery; but then again, you may not feel any symptoms until weeks after you return home. Then you may endure persistent diarrhea, abdominal pain, or indigestion without realizing that it could be the consequence of your trip. Sometimes I see a patient who complains of years of irritable bowel syndrome. When I ask about her travels, I hear about that telltale trip some time ago to Leningrad or to the Taj Mahal. "Oh, I had diarrhea for about a week," this patient tells me, "but then I got better." Yes, but not entirely: a case of amebiasis remained undetected.

Sometimes people who are studying or working abroad for extended periods find that even when they take precautions, they have diarrhea for about two weeks to a month when they first arrive. Mexican travelers visiting the United States are often as uncomfortable as Americans suffering from "Montezuma's revenge." These people's problem is not necessarily harmful microorganisms, just unfamiliar ones. After they've settled down in their adopted home, their diarrhea stops: their guts seem to adjust, although they should still take precautions. If they move again to another country, they often go through the same process all over again.

Your digestive tract *can* accommodate itself to a new environment. For example, the intestinal flora of hospital patients changes within only a few days of their admission to reflect the hospital's flora. This is not very good news when you consider what can turn up in hospitals and the high incidence of illnesses that are actually caused by medical treatment. A study done in India polled natives about their digestion, and then tested them for parasites. Those who had numerous, chronic digestive symptoms turned out to have fewer parasites, while those who had infrequent indigestion or diarrhea harbored more varieties and a higher number of parasites! One way or another, these Indians' gastrointestinal tracts had adapted to their habitat. For *Americans* who had not lived in India all their lives, however, the story would be very different. Their first encounter with Indian parasites would be troublesome.

If a parasitic infection goes undetected and isn't treated, you may suffer from prolonged insidious intestinal illness. Poor nutrition can leave you even more susceptible to parasites. And their irritating presence in your small intestine can make food allergies worse. If you think you have food allergies, make sure that your doctor checks you for parasites as well. Later on in this section on Week Six of the Hoffman Program, I'll be telling you about new methods of detection and treatment for both *Giardia* and amebic infections.

• **Your Pets:** According to veterinarian John Fudens, your pets —cats, dogs, birds—may contract giardiasis, as well as other parasitic infestations, including roundworm, hookworm, *Salmonella*. Birds can have systemic *Candida* infections, while dogs and cats may be infected with *Candida* in their ears or mouth. Animals can also pass bacteria or viruses along to you. In one recent case, a 14-month-old came down with diarrhea and fever that turned out to be signs of infection with bacteria common in tropical fish. As it happened, both the baby and her parents' aquarium had been washed in the same bathtub, allowing the bacteria to pass to the child.

Especially if your pets spend a lot of time outdoors, have them tested regularly for parasites. Even if they never go out, avoid kissing them or letting them lick you or sleep in your bed. Dr. Fudens points out that animals are constantly grooming themselves, and so they can pass fecal bacteria or parasites. Wash your hands carefully if you change a kitty-litter box or clean up after a pup that isn't housebroken yet.

Your Sex

Many women find that their digestion varies with their menstrual cycle: either diarrhea or constipation may accompany menstruation. This is hardly surprising, since your gastrointestinal tract has hormone receptors that make it extremely sensitive to hormonal activity, including that of estrogen and progesterone, which govern the menstrual cycle and pregnancy.

Your digestive tract's sensitivity to these hormones, especially progesterone, is quite obvious when you consider pregnancy's profound effect on digestion. Some pregnant women have heartburn for the first time, because progesterone's activity loosens the esophageal sphincter.

Since your gastrointestinal tract secretes its own hormones, which ensure that all parts of the digestive process take place on time, new findings suggest that gastric hormones in turn affect reproduction. Many expectant mothers feel nauseated, especially during the first trimester, and consequently eat less. Even so, brand-new findings show that gastric hormones ensure that most newly pregnant women gain weight, and continue to do so throughout pregnancy. This wonderfully adaptive mechanism is triggered by increased release of insulin, the hormone that puts fat into cells.

Sometimes diarrhea, lower intestinal bloating, sharp gastric pain, and painful bowel movements during menstruation are signs of endometriosis, a fairly common condition affecting about five million American women with symptoms that range from quite mild to crippling. When you have endometriosis, part of your endometrium, the lining of your uterus, migrates to other parts of your body. There it forms cysts or growths that can be very painful, especially during menstruation, and may block fertility. Endometrial tissue also can imbed itself in the outside walls of your intestines, so that during menstruation your intestinal walls become inflamed. Small wonder you may have intestinal upset and severe pain in your lower abdomen!

Thanks to laser surgery and hormonal treatments, you can get rid of endometrial cysts. But your digestive troubles may not end. As a woman you are more likely to have mitral valve prolapse, a type of heart murmur that is a predominantly female disturbance of the autonomic nervous system, which governs digestion. About fifteen percent of all women have this form of heart murmur, and women who have this physiological peculiarity outnumber men with the same condition by eight to one. Mitral valve prolapse is more than just an isolated anatomical variation affecting the heart; it predisposes you to many kinds of problems involving the autonomic nervous system, including irritable bowel syndrome. Patients with mitral valve prolapse are often given antibiotics during even minor medical and dental procedures to prevent endocarditis. Antibiotics, of course, can leave these patients open to *Candida* infections, which further contribute to any digestive trouble they already have.

The older you are, the more your sex may affect your digestion. Because men have greater body mass and require more protein, they tend to have stronger stomachs, even when they are older. Women, however, have less mass, require less protein, and usually eat lighter food. The result: about 40 percent of women who are over 50 have hypochlorhydria, or a deficiency of stomach acid.

Because lack of stomach acid affects your body's ability to absorb calcium and iron, women of any age who are anemic or have osteoporosis—a condition in which your bones gradually lose minerals and become thin and brittle—generally also have hypochlorhydria. This evidence seems to indicate that your stomach isn't just a passive storage bag for partially digested food; it plays a crucial role in the way your body processes important minerals.

Your Medical and Surgical History

Perhaps you think that because you've had a history of ulcers or acid stomach, you're guaranteed freedom from hypochlorhydria. Not so: low stomach acid may be the sequel to a "burned-out" ulcer. I often see hypochlorhydria in patients who have had severe ulcers in the past.

Constant use of certain drugs, especially remedies for constipation, diarrhea, and acid stomach, but also medications for depression and high blood pressure, may affect your digestive tract's mucosa and the delicate signaling system that allows your gut to set digestive processes in motion at just the right time. With your parents' or your relatives' help, try to list all your childhood illnesses or conditions for which doctors have given you prescriptions. And from now on, if you ever need prolonged medical treatment, keep a log of the drugs you take. Start similar records for your children.

If you've ever been treated for acne, bronchitis, urinary tract or vaginal infections, you may have been given antibiotics. Besides disturbing your intestinal flora and giving you gastric trouble, antibiotics can leave you more vulnerable to *Salmonella*. So do antacids: if you travel abroad while you're on antacids, you run a higher risk of falling prey to bacterial or parasitic infections because your stomach is less acid. Hydrochloric acid is your stomach's best defense against invading pathogens. But antacids can reduce your defense—to the point where it can be breached.

Any form of surgery—even a minor operation like having a wisdom tooth or your tonsils out—may involve doses of antibiotics, and consequently potential gastric trouble. When you actually have gastrointestinal surgery, the effects on your digestion can be drastic. One form of surgery, gastrectomy, which involves removal of all or part of your stomach, used to be a standard part of ulcer treatment. Today, thanks to ulcer drugs, it is very rarely performed.

That's just as well: gastrectomy usually leaves a patient with a condition called "dumping syndrome." Dumping syndrome used to be artificially induced with small-intestine bypass, the very worst form of surgery for the severely overweight. Thank heavens, this drastic option is no longer in vogue. Patients may have lost weight, but they had to endure some gruesome side effects. When you have had a gastrectomy, your stomach's pouch is no longer there to receive your meal. So food moves much too rapidly through your abbreviated gastrointestinal tract to be absorbed properly. You feel as though "dinner ran right through me," especially if you consumed a large quantity of starches, sugars, alcohol, and coffee. A big meal that's heavy in carbohydrates—a pasta dish, perhaps—followed by a sugary dessert like Italian pastries or zabaglione, washed down with wine and espresso, can leave you with all the symptoms of hypoglycemia—flushed face, sweaty palms, and dizziness. As nutrients wash too rapidly through your gut, you also experience nausea and diarrhea. One solution is to eat small meals and to stay away from high-carbohydrate dishes and sugar. Soluble fiber in the form of pectin or guar tablets can help slow your food's journey and aid absorption, because it combines with nutrients so that they work in time-release fashion.

As recently as 1986, another form of gastrointestinal surgery, gastroplasty, was known as "the most popular procedure among surgeons in the United States." But it probably never should have been performed at all, and thankfully it has fallen out of fashion. Meant to be an extreme measure in cases of severe obesity, gastroplasty involves shrinking the stomach by stapling off part of it, creating a small pouch. Another questionable procedure, the gastric balloon, which is no longer an approved procedure, was also used to block off part of the stomach by inserting a small inflated balloon. In theory, both the gastric pouch and balloon helped patients eat less and lose weight more easily and rapidly because they felt full sooner. In fact, neither gastroplasty nor the gastric balloon combated obese patients' primary problem, a compulsion to overeat. Over half of gastroplasty patients didn't lose weight after their surgery, and more than 10 percent suffered major complications besides. The gastric balloon also could lead to various complications, including intestinal blockage and ulcers. And it seemed to be no more effective than a diet in taking weight off.

Two other types of gastrointestinal surgery may be medically necessary. Many patients with colitis or colon cancer eventually require a colectomy, which removes part or all of your large intestine. After your operation, wastes drain directly out of your body, through an incision (a colostomy) in your lower abdomen, down a plastic tube into a plastic bag. Since a major function of your colon is to remove water from digested food, your stool will be more copious after a colectomy. You may also require nutritional supplements to replace the nutrients that your colon used to absorb.

Finally, you may be obliged to have part of your small intestine removed—what is known as a small-intestine bypass. This can be the unfortunate consequence of a bad case of Crohn's disease. Like ulcerative colitis, Crohn's disease is a serious form of inflammatory bowel disease. But while ulcerative colitis affects only your large intestine, Crohn's disease can make itself felt anywhere from your mouth to your anus, but it usually affects your small intestine. If you must have small-intestine surgery, the nutritional consequences are much worse than they are after a colectomy. Because your small intestine absorbs so many important nutrients, you may end up with short-gut syndrome, an extreme form of malabsorption.

When you have short-gut syndrome, you have trouble absorbing fat, and hence frequent attacks of fatty diarrhea. If you are unable to absorb fat, you cannot absorb fat-soluble vitamins, including A, D, E, and K, as well as certain essential fatty acids. Vitamin A deficiency may lead to night blindness. Another common side effect of this inability to absorb fats is kidney stones. As fats pass through you, they bind with calcium and form too much oxalic acid, which hardens into kidney stones. When you pass kidney stones, you can feel excruciating pain—and may end up with a damaged urinary tract.

If you are obliged to have your entire small intestine removed, you cannot live without hyperalimentation—a formula full of essential nutrients infused intravenously. Researchers discovered that trace elements like selenium and chromium were crucial to human nutrition because, without infusions, patients began to waste away. The efficiency of the small intestine is clear when you consider the fact that, without it, an infusion that lasts about fourteen hours has to replace a normal meal. Since you have to remain tethered to an IV during your infusion, your life is severely limited.

Staying Well-Fed While You Get Well

While gastrointestinal surgery can have particularly devastating effects on your digestion, any major surgery can leave you malnourished, especially if you have to be fed intravenously afterward. At least one to three weeks before surgery, you should begin taking nutritional supplements to counteract any temporary malabsorption or malnutrition. You should be especially careful to eat meals rich in protein, vitamins A, C, E, B_1, B_2, B_5, B_{12} (these B vitamins are plentiful in organ meats and brewer's yeast), folic acid (found in leafy greens), and the minerals zinc, iron, potassium, magnesium, and selenium. I also recommend a high-potency multivitamin, a multimineral, and extra vitamin E, vitamin C, and potassium, along with acidophilus to ward off digestion problems.

Cancer, especially gastric cancer, is a particular drain on your body's nutrients. If you vomit or lose your appetite after chemotherapy, you will have more trouble staying adequately nourished—a prime requisite for healing and avoiding complications.

There is one final way that your medical condition can affect your digestion: if your immune system has been weakened, you are especially vulnerable to parasites and foodborne infections. If you think you are at risk, either because you are susceptible to infections or because you're under stress, ask your nutritionally oriented doctor for a salivary IGA test. This simple office procedure can determine the strength of your gastrointestinal immune system. If your immune system has been seriously compromised by chemotherapy or an illness like AIDS, you'd be wise to pass up salad bars. When you go to a delicatessen or restaurant, avoid raw food and sandwiches or salads with mayonnaise, which may contain *Salmonella*. If you're obliged to travel, you must take special precautions, as I outlined in the previous section.

Your Diet

Bad habits like excessive alcohol, smoking, and too many nitrates, nitrites, and other preservatives can put you on a four-lane highway to gastric trouble. A history of haphazard eating habits (perhaps due to a job that keeps you constantly on the road or has irregular hours), sudden radical changes in diet (thanks to crash dieting or eating disorders like anorexia or bulimia), or overeating can predispose you to digestion problems.

But it's quite possible to err in the other direction—to be so conscientious about dieting or about consuming natural food that your digestion suffers. If you are on a diet, have been careful to eat dietetic foods, and have been plagued by frequent attacks of diarrhea, check the labels on your diet brands. They may contain sorbitol or xylitol, sweeteners that can't be absorbed and that might be upsetting your stomach.

If you have irritable bowel syndrome, or some other gastric trouble that can flare up under stress, perhaps you've stocked up on chamomile tea. This particular herb tea is indeed calming, but it is also constipating. If you tend to be constipated anyway, switch to passion flower tea when you need something soothing. Peppermint tea is another herbal remedy for irritable bowel syndrome and gastric upset. But it is useless if you have heartburn—in fact, peppermint tea will make reflux worse. Try aloe vera or licorice or comfrey tea instead. But go easy on the latter two: studies have shown that licorice can contribute to hypertension, while steady consumption of comfrey tea can lead to liver disease.

Similarly, if you try to cure a cold with too frequent, too heavy doses of vitamin C, it may give you diarrhea. If you make sure you're getting enough calcium by overdosing on calcium carbonate, you may find you're constipated. Bear in mind that calcium carbonate, which many people take in the form of Tums, is the same substance that makes up the White Cliffs of Dover! By taking too much calcium carbonate, you may be petrifying your gut. Switch to calcium citrate, which is not binding.

If you are too conscientious about your fiber intake, you may overdose. One 64-year-old doctor was not immune: he worked at a hospital that had begun serving highly potent bran muffins—a pleasant surprise considering the generally abysmal reputation of most hospital food. This doctor knew the value of fiber: for years, he had been eating salads almost every day, as well as a high-fiber breakfast cereal. Naturally, he thought the muffins were a fine addition to his good diet. He had never had intestinal problems before, but suddenly he was suffering from gas, cramping, and explosive diarrhea two or three times a day.

Luckily he happened to consult another physician who was even better educated than he was about nutrition. This man took a detailed history of his patient's dietary habits. The bran muffins had dramatically increased his fiber intake, which had been already at a healthful level. His doctor prescribed giving up the hospital's muffins, and within the next two to three days, the patient's bowel movements returned to normal, and remained so. With oat-bran mania at its peak, I certainly hope that millions of Americans are not duplicating his experience.

Looking Over Your Body

Like the way you've been living, your body can give you many hints and clues to the nature of your digestive troubles. Take a good look at yourself from head to toe.

• *Your Hair:* If your hair is dry and brittle, frequently breaking off so that your hairdresser has to snip off all your "split ends," you're deficient in certain vitamins, minerals, essential fatty acids or amino acids—classic signs of malabsorption. Other clues that point to nutrient deficiency are dry skin and nails that break or peel easily.

• *Your Forehead:* Dull headaches at your temples often accompany chronic constipation. Significantly, *hegu,* the most effective acupuncture pressure point for headaches, is a spot between your thumb and forefinger that is on the same meridian—a system of alignment in Chinese medicine—as your colon. If you eradicate a digestive problem, your headaches often disappear as well.

• *Your Eyes:* Night blindness, along with kidney stones, anemia and osteoporosis, is a sign of malabsorption as an aftereffect of gastrointestinal surgery.

• *Your Tongue:* According to Chinese medical tradition, your tongue mirrors your internal condition. There are literally hundreds of different ways the tongue can look—each corresponding to a certain state of illness or health. But generally speaking, if you're feeling well, your tongue is pink and smooth. If you're run-down or ill, your tongue may be yellow or look creamy. A coated tongue usually is a sign of poor digestion.

• *Your Lower Lip:* Chinese medicine also considers your face an important diagnostic tool. A red and swollen lower lip may correspond to poor intestinal tone—a swelling of your large intestine, which may be inflamed as well. Cracks in your lower lip can indicate a full-blown case of colitis.

• *Your Teeth:* If your teeth are grayish, you may have taken large doses of tetracycline as a child, while your teeth were still developing. Your digestive problems, then, may be side effects of antibiotics. Check your medical history for the kinds of prescriptions you've been given over the years.

• *Your Breath:* If you have chronic bad breath, first make appointments for checkups with your dentist and with an ear, nose, and throat specialist as well. If they rule out tooth or gum disease, along with sinus or nasal infection, your problem is more than a social handicap: it may be due to reflux or lack of hydrochloric acid. Because your stomach acid is low, food may be putrefying instead of breaking down inside you. By taking supplemental hydrochloric acid, you can easily overcome this stasis. Bad breath may also mean you are infected with *Campylobacter pylori*, the bacteria that cause ulcers.

Once a patient came to me complaining of chronic bad breath. She had found mouthwash ineffective, and other doctors had dismissed her problem. Since I suspected the presence of a bacterial infection, I gave my patient supplemental doses of hydrochloric acid. When her bad breath persisted, I sent her to a gastroenterologist, suggesting a test for *C. pylori*. He confirmed my suspicions, so I tried giving her a course of Pepto-Bismol to combat *C. pylori*, and her bad breath cleared up. Her infection had not yet progressed far enough to give her an ulcer; her bad breath, caused by her infection, was the only clue to what was really wrong.

• *Your Mouth and Throat:* When you eat, do you feel "as though my food has stuck in my craw"? Can you taste your meal for hours afterward? These sensations may indicate that you lack stomach acid.

• *Your Belly:* If, on the other hand, you're in pain when your stomach is empty, and feel relief after you eat something, you may have too much stomach acid, or an ulcer.

Another stomach clue is excessive bloating, which can point to an intestinal *Candida* infection. Once a patient told me, "Whenever I eat, my stomach literally sticks out as if I were pregnant." I must have looked dubious, because she added, "You think I'm kidding?" and laid several before-and-after-dinner snapshots on my desk. She hadn't exaggerated: thanks to *Candida*'s fermenting action, her gut was producing so much intestinal gas that after a meal, her stomach rose like bread.

Your Window on Your Own Digestion

The best external clues that your body can provide to what's going on inside you are your feces. Observing your own stool gives you the widest, clearest view you can have of your own digestion. In fact, anthropologists have studied fossilized human feces, called coprolites, to find out what our ancestors could and couldn't digest. Amazingly, when scientists soak coprolites in powerful detergent to soften them and make them easier to study, coprolites smell as pungent as they must have on a warm day six thousand years ago. How's that for reliving ancient history!

Your stool's weight, consistency, color, and so on are important diagnostic tools: they can tell you and your doctor quite a bit about the state of your digestive tract. Now, it's quite natural to be interested in your own stool. Producing one was probably your very first creative act, and among your most applauded. But there's a difference between being aware of your bowel movements and being obsessed with them. Some avid stool readers go overboard and assume that any small fluctuation merits a call to their doctor, especially if they think they are constipated. In my experience, such people often suffer from other forms of performance anxiety.

Judging by television advertising, most Americans are preoccupied with being regular. But how regular is regular? Some colon-health enthusiasts and advocates of colonics and other forms of colon therapy believe that your system isn't cleansing itself properly unless you have at least two movements a day, one in the morning and one later on. On the other hand, some conventionally trained physicians don't necessarily consider daily movements, or movements that occur at the same times every day, a sign of good health.

During my second year of medical school, I attended an unusually crowded lecture entitled "Diarrhea and Constipation." By this point in my studies, the throngs of lecture-goers had thinned considerably, because many students had adopted a stay-at-home study plan. But the alluring title of this talk packed them in. The expert started out by asking us, "Who do you think is better off—a patient who has a bowel movement twice a day, or one who has a bowel movement twice a week?"

The answer, he said, is that neither is better off, because there is no such thing as optimal bowel habits, only individual patterns. A better definition of constipation, then, is longer intervals between movements than is normal *for you.*

Well, I disagreed with the expert, and still do. He was teaching a generation of future doctors to ignore the lessons British researcher Dr. Denis P. Burkitt had already gleaned during his sojourn in rural Africa, where people eliminate dietary waste in about one-third the time we do, concerning the benefits of a fibrous diet. It *is* better to have two or more bowel movements a day. Rapid transit is a hedge against diverticulosis, colon cancer, and other diseases of civilization. British physician Hugh C. Trowell, who along with Burkitt coined the phrase "dietary fiber" in 1976, has since speculated that one reason fiber eaters have colon cancer less often is that the carcinogens they ingest with their food speed out of their bodies, as fiber accelerates their transit time.

On the other hand, I certainly don't regard an obsession with regularity or with your feces generally as a sign of good physical or psychological health. But feces certainly do mirror the way you live, and can be read like tea leaves—to decipher your present digestive health and foretell its future. You can use your feces to spot digestive problems, and to figure out what you need to do to treat and prevent them. Here are the clues you should be looking for in your toilet bowl.

• **Transit Time:** An important clue is your transit time, the interval between the moment you swallow a mouthful and the moment you excrete the waste that remains after digestion is complete. For a week before your appointment with your doctor, keep a feces diary, just as you've been keeping a diet diary. This will help you figure out what "normal" and "regular" means for your own gastrointestinal tract. For each 24-hour period, note how many bowel movements you have, and the times at which they occurred.

Transit time is highly individual, but if yours is 18 hours or less, you may be suffering from malabsorption. Without adequate breakdown and assimilation, even the healthiest meals are of little benefit to your body. On the other hand, a transit time that's longer than 72 hours may be equally unhealthy. Dr. Denis Burkitt has suggested that slow transit, which is very common in industrialized countries, can predispose you to chronic digestive illness. The longer your transit time, the longer waste products can linger inside you and create unhealthy conditions.

You can test your own transit time by using charcoal tablets, sold in most health-food stores and drugstores as a remedy for intestinal gas. Right after you have a bowel movement, take 20 grams of charcoal (about 5–10 tablets, depending on their size), and note the time you swallow them. When you have your next bowel movement, note again how long it takes before you see black stool. When charcoal appears as black stool in your toilet bowl, your home test is complete, and you have a rough notion of your average transit time. Less than 18 hours probably means you are not absorbing nutrients properly; more than 72 hours means that food may sit in your gut, leaving you at risk for serious intestinal illness.

Besides transit time, there are some other important characteristics of your feces that you should keep track of in your week-long diary.

• *Color:* Your feces' normal color is brown because colonic bacteria make brown pigments out of bile that your liver secretes into your small intestine to help you absorb fats. Although your feces do change in appearance from day to day, only dramatic, lasting shifts in color are potentially important. For example, your feces may be red or black for a day because you consumed a generous portion of beets, meat, chocolate, Hydrox cookies, licorice, cherries, or even over-the-counter remedies like Pepto-Bismol or iron pills. But if your stool remains consistently black, you may have bleeding in your upper gastrointestinal tract. Occasional bloody streaks on the outside of your stool may come from hemorrhoids or temporary anal irritation. If blood appears persistently, and appears to be mixed into your stool, your lower gastrointestinal tract may be bleeding. In either case, you need to see your doctor.

Unless you have been eating foods high in chlorophyll, a yellow or greenish stool is usually a sign of diarrhea and transit time that is too rapid. If you are taking antibiotics, this color may mean that your bowel has been sterilized. A tan or clay color may indicate that you have eaten too much fat, or that your bile duct is blocked and is not producing enough bile to digest normal amounts of fat. Finally, a yellowish hue may be a sign that your pancreas is not producing enough digestive enzymes. If your stool turns almost white, the culprit may be antacids or excess calcium supplements.

• **Consistency:** A normal stool has a distinct sausagelike shape, but is soft and plastic. Variations may occur from day to day if you have mild diarrhea, constipation, or protein malabsorption, or if you occasionally binge on a favorite food.

A small, dry stool that sinks to the bottom of your toilet bowl indicates a diet that is too high in meat. But a floating stool is not always a sign of a diet with plenty of fiber, rapid transit time, and general digestive health. A stool that floats but is too loose is a sign of diarrhea and, consequently, malabsorption—perhaps due to irritable bowel syndrome. Narrow, ribbonlike stools are a common clue to irritable bowel syndrome, or even a partial obstruction in your intestinal tract that might be an early warning sign of cancer. Stools that float but are voluminous, pasty, and greasy, leaving an oil slick on the surface of the water in your toilet, may mean that you're eating too much fat, or that you are having trouble absorbing fat normally because enzyme production has declined. This type of stool also may be a sign of celiac sprue or pancreatitis.

You should be able to see only a very few undigested food particles or fibers in your stool. If you spot a substantial number, you may not be chewing your food thoroughly enough. Or you may lack crucial digestive enzymes. Undigested meat cells or vegetable fibers, sometimes visible only under your doctor's microscope, are a sign of insufficient hydrochloric acid or pancreatic enzyme production, something that interferes with protein absorption.

You also should not see any mucus or pus in your stool. The presence of mucus may indicate that you have irritable bowel syndrome, food allergies, or an inflammation of your intestinal wall, possibly thanks to a parasitic or *Candida* infection. Pus may be a warning sign of diverticulitis or parasites. If you have diarrhea with both mucus and pus, your trouble may be ulcerative colitis or a parasitic infection. Bloody diarrhea accompanied by mucus can mean colitis or Crohn's disease.

But if you spot a little fleck of blood in or around your stool now and then, don't panic. It is *not* necessarily a sign of colon cancer or an ulcer. A few spots can herald cancer, but if you have a serious ulcer, you would bleed much more rapidly and noticeably, and you would feel faint. Occasional specks of blood are probably due to hemorrhoids or anal fissures, but do ask your doctor to check. The presence of blood in your stool can also indicate colitis or parasitic infection.

• *Smell: A False Clue:* A popular myth among advocates of colonics and colon health is that a healthy stool has no smell. In fact, there is no such thing as an odorless stool. Meat eaters do tend to have more odoriferous stools because protein may yield residues of nitrogen and sulfur, but it is neither possible nor desirable to eliminate odor from stool.

In Your Doctor's Office

You have now learned just about all you can by observing your stools and your body with the only tool you have, your naked eye. If you suspect malabsorption or have a chronic complaint, you need to take a specimen of your stool to a doctor who will examine it more completely under a microscope and analyze its contents. Now, even though this test, known as the comprehensive digestive stool analysis (CDSA), is one of the most important of all diagnostic tools for digestive disorders, at present it is not usually part of a conventional checkup. Doctors are apt to bypass it in favor of putting a scope up or down your gut—an invasive, expensive, and sometimes risky procedure. To make sure you can get a stool analysis, make an appointment with a progressive internist or gastroenterologist, or a nutritionally oriented doctor.

But even the most forward-thinking doctor can't test you for fat malabsorption if you have eaten no fat. For two or three days before you plan to see your doctor about your gastrointestinal problems, your diet should include protein (eggs, whole grains, meat, fish), vegetables, starch (rice, potatoes, sweet potatoes, bread), and fat (butter and oil). Your doctor will probably tell you in advance how and when to collect your stool sample, usually the morning of the day of your appointment.

Take along with you to your appointment your food diary and your feces diary, as well as any additional notes you have taken on your gastrointestinal symptoms and the appearance of your stool. Your doctor will certainly take blood and stool specimens, but there may be some special tests you will want to request, depending on the results he or she gets.

Your Stool Analysis: What It Can Detect

A microscopic stool analysis will look in more detail for some of the same signs that you have checked for: the presence of undigested food particles, mucus, blood, or pus in your feces. Meat cells and vegetable fibers are important signs of low stomach acid and weak enzyme production. This examination will also determine whether the amounts of starch, fat and fatty acids in your stool are within normal levels. An elevated level of any of these substances may indicate that you lack bile or pancreatic enzymes.

Microbiological analysis of your stool specimen can determine whether friendly bacteria are present in normal quantities, whether you have a yeast overgrowth, and whether there is any bile in your stool. If there is bile, your transit time is much too rapid, and you may have a food allergy or some other cause of diarrhea. An elevated level of fats may indicate that you're deficient in pancreatic enzymes. This test will also determine the alkalinity of your stool. Too much indicates low stomach acid, an imbalance of bowel flora, or possibly transit time that is too rapid because of food allergies or even eating too much fiber. On the other hand, too little alkalinity may indicate that you have been eating a great deal of meat, or it may mean insufficient pancreatic enzymes.

Chemical analysis will also check for occult blood—meaning blood that is invisible to your naked eye—in your stool. This may be inconsequential, the result of hemorrhoids or a meal of raw or very rare meat. Or it may be a warning sign of colon cancer. In medicine, we continually discuss how to spot colon cancer early without putting patients through endless expensive tests that may turn out to be unnecessary. In the early 1980s, when Dr. Russell Jaffe, then at the National Institutes of Health, invented the Hemoccult test, it was considered a breakthrough in colon-cancer testing because it was so easy and inexpensive. Patients could perform it by themselves at home, without going to the doctor for feces analysis to check for occult blood. You simply wiped yourself with toilet paper, dabbed the paper on a special card, and mailed the card to your doctor. The doctor then exposed the card to a developer. If the card turned a bluish color, your test was positive, and further investigation for signs of cancer would be warranted.

But this card test turned out to be something less than hoped for, because it can be confounded by high levels of iron in your stool thanks to bleeding from hemorrhoids, or your diet. Vitamin C supplements can also invalidate test results. There have been so many false-positives, engendering so many needless colonoscopies—an invasive, elaborate, and occasionally hazardous test to detect colon cancer—that some doctors no longer recommend the Hemoccult test for routine screening. If your family's medical history or your previous illnesses indicate that you are particularly at risk, and ought to take the Hemoccult test, make sure that your doctor instructs you carefully about foods and vitamins to avoid, lest they skew your test results. New tests are in the works, but to date, no fail-safe colon cancer test exists.

If Your Problem Is Something Other Than Cancer

Unless you need further tests to make sure you don't have colon cancer, here are some typical patterns that might emerge from your doctor's analysis of your stool. If you have high alkalinity, undigested food particles, or other signs of low stomach acid, a nutritionally oriented doctor will probably recommend a Heidelberg test, which is really a more sophisticated version of the charcoal test you did at home.

Part of the reason why digestive malabsorption due to low stomach acid or decreased secretion of pancreatic enzymes has been often overlooked is that, until recently, effective and simple tests were not available. Determining your gastrointestinal pH, a measure of acidity and alkalinity, gives me a great deal of information about your digestion. For normal digestion, your stomach should be sufficiently acid and your small intestine on the alkaline side. As your food exits your stomach and enters your small intestine, it has to be acidic enough to trigger the proper release of pancreatic enzymes, which work best in an alkaline environment. If your stomach is not acidic enough, your small intestine is likely to be overly acidic. Enzymes won't be released, and nutrients won't be absorbed.

The old-fashioned way of measuring gastrointestinal acidity involved inserting a tube through your nose into your gut. Besides being unpleasant, this procedure only measured stomach acidity. But a new test developed at the University of Heidelberg, in Germany, measures small-intestinal acidity as well.

The Heidelberg test involves swallowing a small indigestible capsule containing a radio transmitter. A technician then monitors its reading of the pH of your gastrointestinal tract. As it passes through your gastrointestinal tract, the capsule also measures your transit time for the early phases of digestion.

If you are low in hydrochloric acid, you can take it in supplements for three to six months. Surprisingly, your digestion doesn't start depending on this extra boost; rather, the supplements often give your gut a chance to rest and regenerate itself. Supplementing your diet with specific nutrients will also help, especially folic acid, which is vital to secretion of hydrochloric acid.

Enzyme Tests

When your stool contains a high level of fat and undigested vegetable particles or meat cells, you may have low enzyme production, due to lack of stomach acid or some other cause. I might order a Chymex test, which measures digestive residues in your urine. Hair analysis can also provide clues: low levels of essential minerals like zinc, manganese, copper, chromium, and selenium may indicate low stomach acid and attendant low enzyme production.

If you lack the enzymes you need, you can take supplements, which work best if crushed or granulated and taken with your meals. They do have an unpleasant taste, however, so you may prefer to take enteric-coated capsules—coated so that they are released past your stomach—which are slightly less effective but more palatable.

Parasites: A Medical Detective's Challenge

Microbiological analysis of your stool specimen is not the gold standard in one particular area: detecting parasites and their eggs, which may not necessarily show up under the microscope.

The two most common kinds of parasitic infection worldwide are caused by *Giardia* and amoebas. Although *Giardia* resides in your jejunum, the upper portion of your small intestine, while amoebas generally live lower down in your gut, these two parasites have some common characteristics. Both can cause immediate, strong symptoms —explosive diarrhea, severe cramping—that alert you that something is obviously very wrong with your gut. Both *Giardia* and amoebas may also instigate minor, inconsequential discomfort that comes and goes over time and that you may not recognize as a sign of insidious parasitic infection. Once diagnosed, *Giardia* and amoebas can be treated similarly. But both pose a considerable diagnostic challenge to a medical detective.

Because you excrete parasites only intermittently, and then sometimes in very small quantities, the organisms don't show up under the microscope in the stool specimens of as many as half of infected patients. To try to detect parasites, doctors used to ask for and analyze several stool samples over a period of time. But even with conscientious retrials, stool analysis is not foolproof. If you analyze one stool specimen, you have a 40 percent chance of detecting parasites. If you analyze a second specimen as well, your chances rise to 60 percent. And if you do a third analysis, your chances become 70 percent—still leaving a substantial margin of diagnostic error.

Actually, it makes good sense that parasites don't often show up in stool. Unlike bacteria in your large intestine, they don't thrive on feces. Rather, they try to adhere to and suck blood from your intestinal walls. So they are much less likely to appear in stool, but they might show up right next to your intestinal walls, in the blanket of mucus that covers them. The most efficient way to detect parasites, I think, is to obtain a sample of that mucus.

If I suspect parasitic infection, I generally recommend a new, painless test, the rectal swab test, which is much simpler and more accurate than repeated stool analyses. Using a small plastic anoscope, your doctor inserts a cotton swab into your anus and daubs vigorously to obtain one or more specimens of mucus from the walls of your large intestine. When the sample is analyzed, highly sensitive stains light up with traces of parasite debris, confirming the presence of amoebas, *Giardia*, or other bugs. Since *Candida* often coexists with parasites, ask your doctor to take a separate mucus sample to check for a yeast infection.

I have already mentioned the CDSA, a test that provides information that a rectal mucus swab can't. The CDSA tells your doctor the precise mix of bacteria in your intestinal flora, and so it is a fine way to check for *Candida* and to monitor the general health of your flora. But this test is not an especially reliable way to find parasites: it picks up only those that have shed off your intestinal walls into your stool. But since the CDSA test detects bacterial overgrowth, it complements the mucus swab test nicely. I often recommend both tests for patients with persistent bowel problems.

Double-Checking for Giardia

Sometimes a patient who has had a mucus swab that appeared clean of parasites under the microscope still has symptoms of giardiasis. Since an anoscope doesn't penetrate very far into your colon to take a mucus swab, this test could miss *Giardia*, since it lives in the jejunum, the upper portion of your small intestine. If I suspect *Giardia*, but have found a clean mucus swab, I have to consider some more complicated tests specifically for this parasite.

A jejunal biopsy, which has to be done with an endoscopy, through the upper part of your intestine, can find *Giardia*. But this test is difficult to perform, hard on the patient, and expensive to boot. It can be a last resort, but there is an effective and cheaper alternative: "fishing" for *Giardia* in the jejunum.

This test, called the Enterotest, works like this: at home, just before bedtime, you take a gelatin capsule with nylon yarn packed inside, with a tiny hidden lead weight (covered in rubber to prevent lead poisoning) at the very end of the yarn. The other end of the yarn is loose and sticks out of the capsule, like the end of a spool of thread. You tape this loose end of the yarn to your cheek, and then you swallow the capsule. Over the next few hours, the capsule dissolves, and almost five feet of nylon yarn unravel and stretch through your duodenum and jejunum. The next morning, you pull the yarn back up through your mouth; as you do, the lead weight drops off, to be safely excreted eventually. The yarn is now covered with mucus and bile. This can be examined under the microscope, which should reveal *Giardia*'s presence.

Chasing Parasites Out

Once you are sure you have a parasite, the best remedy may be an immediate, powerful dose of antibiotics. But some have terrible side effects: Quinacrine, most doctors' drug of choice for giardiasis, can trigger mental instability—even psychosis—and it can turn your complexion yellow. Flagyl, the drug prescribed most often for amoebas, may make you nauseous, give you diarrhea, and leave an awful metallic taste in your mouth. If you take Flagyl and then drink alcohol, you may become severely ill.

All too often, these drugs not only prove ineffectual but aggravate intestinal imbalance because they strip your large intestine of its friendly flora. Frequently, I see patients who have already undergone multiple rounds of antiparasitic drug therapy, but who feel no improvement in their gastrointestinal complaints, fatigue, and malaise. At that point, I have to wonder whether the problem is still the parasites or the devastating effects of the drugs themselves, which have acted like chemical defoliants, denuding these patients' intestinal landscape.

Instead of prescribing drugs, I suggest that because parasites thrive on carbohydrates, patients should limit their intake, especially in the form of wheat and dairy products, sugar, fruits and fruit juices. Meanwhile, they can foster their normal intestinal flora by taking acidophilus and hydrochloric acid.

What if parasites are still lurking? Garlic (especially in the form of deodorized capsules that do not affect your breath), pumpkin seeds, and black walnut extract are excellent, time-tested enemies of parasites. Recently, some new herbal medications have been added to my antiparasitic arsenal. My colleague Dr. Leo Galland, a nutritionally oriented physician in New York City with a particular interest in parasites, reports good results with patients who have taken an active form of artemisia (or wormwood) and a special extract of grapefruit seed once used by Amazon Indians.

Week Seven:
Change
Your Style

*"A reliable set of bowels is worth more to a man than any quantity
of brains."*

—*Henry Wheeler Shaw,*
nineteenth-century humorist

This week, I'm going to show you how a conscious attempt to
consider exactly *how* you eat—and then changing it—can improve
your digestion. I'm also going to point out some new ways of thinking
about your digestive tract and how it works. These can guide you
toward types of treatment that you may not have realized could help
you.

Think About It: Do You Fall
for Food Fallacies?

A quick glance around any bookstore brings home how interested
modern Americans are in nutrition and diet. Of course, I'm delighted
that people are taking the link between health and diet more seriously.
But watch out! There are diets and food plans that make extravagant
or spurious promises about the virtues of their particular approaches.

Because food is essential to life and health, many cultures throughout history have not been able to resist endowing it with potent significance. Today, thanks to science and medicine, we know much more about food's real properties than ancient peoples did. But enough controversy continues over scientific evidence that there's still room for food folklore—beliefs that endow certain foods or diets with potent properties, and that usually reflect real ignorance of how your physiology works during digestion. Food folklore can give rise to food fallacies.

For example, sometimes I see people who are obviously quite ill—they're suffering from fatigue, bloating, painful gas, and they have foul-smelling stools. Frequently they are emaciated, with dry hair and skin. When I question these people, I discover that their main concern is "detoxification"; in an attempt to purify themselves, they have decided to eat only fruits and vegetables, or only lichens, or, in one case, only vegetable juices. They are convinced that they are ill because, despite their regimens, they have eaten the wrong food; if they just detox some more, they will regain their health.

What's actually happened is that these people have detoxed to the point of illness, and their bodies are breaking down. The proof is the fact that if they try to eat a range of foods, they cannot tolerate them. When you are malnourished, you lose digestive enzymes, especially those that help you break down proteins. But these poor deluded individuals believe that their increasing food intolerances are nature's way of flagging their extensive "food allergies."

Another recent example of a popular food fallacy was starch blockers. Thankfully, the Federal Food and Drug Administration has regulated promotion of this dubious product—one of the very few instances where I'm in complete agreement with the FDA! Basically, starch blockers are a purified version of a substance that beans contain to hinder your digesting them. That way, they can pass out of you almost intact—evolution's way of ensuring that undigested beans might fall into soil and sprout into new beans. In principle, then, starch blockers are supposed to prevent your digesting carbohydrates, thereby helping you lose weight.

Unfortunately, this principle just doesn't work in practice. Not only do dieters who take starch blockers experience terrible indigestion and uncomfortable bloating, but their absorption of carbohydrates is almost identical with that of people who pass up starch blockers.

Some food fallacies contain a kernel of truth. One example is the theory of food combining, promoted by the very popular Fit for Life diet. Food combining has its roots in the theories of Sylvester Graham, the graham cracker's namesake. Graham was a nineteenth-century "back-to-nature" health reformer who was rightly suspicious of processed foods. Nutritionist Herbert M. Shelton, a Graham acolyte who died in 1985 at the age of 89, took Graham's thinking one step further: Shelton advised his patients against eating more than one type of food at a single meal. He believed that "eating wrong combinations of foods" is "one of the most common causes of digestive inefficiency." Moreover, he claimed that if you eat during illness, your meals will putrefy inside you instead of being digested. And he advocated regular fasting, especially during illness, to eliminate that rotting food.

While Shelton had some sensible ideas, like "a salad a day" for all ages, he badly misconstrued the nature of digestion, especially the role of enzymes. "Each enzyme is specific in its action," Shelton wrote. "That is to say, it acts only upon one class of food substance." It's quite true that there are different types of enzymes that work on different foods, but Shelton went on to claim that your digestive enzymes were capable of breaking down only one sort of foodstuff at a time—a complete misinterpretation of the digestive process. Digestive enzymes go to work when they are needed. They can work on proteins, fats, and carbohydrates simultaneously, and don't have to wait their turn.

Shelton was also wrong about putrefaction—which was a common misconception of how food is absorbed before physiologists understood the digestive process. Some fermentation does occur in your intestines, as a natural and desirable part of digestion. If you haven't been eating enough fiber, food may be moving sluggishly through your digestive tract. But rarely will anything putrefy, as Shelton warned; "putrefaction" is actually the natural process of food being broken down with the help of bacteria.

Many of Shelton's woeful misconceptions survived in the best-selling Fit for Life diet. Among its strange notions of how digestion works are these: eating foods in the wrong combinations means that they won't be absorbed, but will ferment and rot inside you, leading to all kinds of illness; some foods "cleanse" your body, while others "clog" it; fruit is a "cleanser," but if you eat it as dessert, it will ferment and won't be absorbed. In fact, the Fit for Life diet says that "fruit should never be eaten with or immediately following anything"

—a rule it calls "unquestionably the most important aspect" of this regimen.

Like Herbert Shelton, its mentor, Fit for Life is shockingly ignorant of the basic functioning of your digestive tract. There is no physiological reason why eating foods in particular combinations should either help or hinder digestion. All food, no matter when or how you eat it, is broken down and mixed together in your stomach. By the time it leaves your stomach as chyme, your careful combinations no longer exist. And when chyme arrives in your small intestine, your digestive enzymes are perfectly capable of going to work all at the same time, breaking down whatever you happen to have eaten.

Strict adherence to the Fit for Life diet can have serious consequences for diabetics, hypoglycemics, the elderly, and women who are pregnant or lactating. However, there are some health benefits to Fit for Life. Its emphasis on fresh, raw fruits and vegetables and their juices, and on avoiding or strictly limiting all animal fats, meat, and dairy products can help you make a habit of eating more fiber and lowering your cholesterol. And although not everyone is obliged to practice food combining, some people seem to digest more comfortably if they adhere to it. This is why avid food-combining enthusiasts exist.

Any fermentation process, whether it takes place in a fermenting vat, in rising dough, or in your stomach, requires a sugar "starter." In your stomach, fermentation breaks down starchy carbohydrates. This is a perfectly normal process that usually doesn't cause digestive discomfort. But for some people, eating starches along with sugar or fruit triggers excessive gas and bloating. If your stomach's fermentation is unduly exacerbated by additional sugar, washing down your favorite vegetable chili with a glass of wine or fruit juice can give you gas and indigestion.

If that's the case, food combining may make sense for you. One food-combining principle that apparently helps alleviate severe flatulence is to eat fruit or drink fruit juice at least a half hour before and two hours after a meal. If you do eat sugary foods, combine them with protein—which doesn't ferment in your stomach—and not with complex carbohydrates. The popular French dessert of fruit and cheese obviously is based on classic food-combining principles. Another good combination is fruit and yogurt. And by all means ignore the advice I saw printed recently on a T-shirt: "Life is uncertain. Eat dessert first."

What will be certain for you is that empty calories will crowd out nutrients.

The Virtues of Fasting

Herbert Shelton was not off base when he wrote that fasting "is a sure means of providing rest for an overworked digestive system." Provided that your overall health is good, an occasional fast is not a food fallacy: it gives your digestive organs a brief break from their nonstop labor of breaking down and absorbing nutrients. Then your body can put more energy into eliminating toxic materials and wastes that are the by-products of your meals. Fasting is an ancient method of purifying yourself physiologically—and spiritually as well. If you've been following the Hoffman Program week by week and have changed your eating habits, now is a good time to fast for a day or so, to allow your body to cleanse itself and heal.

Some of the debates over how and when to fast, along with rules on how to break a fast, make amusing reading. The ultimate food faddist was probably Professor Arnold Ehret, a fasting advocate who theorized that "all disease is finally nothing else but a clogging up of the smallest blood vessels, the capillaries, by mucus." Ehret considered fasting an essential part of his "Mucus-less Diet Healing System"—a fruit diet with a rationale similar to Herbert Shelton's advice on avoiding internal putrefaction. Ehret insisted that drinking broth or juice constituted a liquid diet, not a proper fast: if you were fasting, you should drink only spring water.

I part company with the good professor here. There *is* a system to fasting, but I think that besides spring water, it is fine to drink some diluted vegetable broth or fruit or vegetable juice three or four times daily. You can drink six to eight cups or glasses—just as you normally drink that much water—but don't hesitate to take more if you're thirsty. Some options, such as diluted miso broth, herb teas, carrot juice, or watermelon juice, are delicious. (To make watermelon juice, just put watermelon without seeds into your blender with a little water.) Unless you plan to spend your fast immobile—not a very healthy idea!—you need some nourishment, especially if you want to regenerate damaged parts of your digestive tract. You can certainly work and exercise; long walks are fine. I've found that if I try really strenuous aerobic exercise while fasting, I have stamina but not much strength. When you break your fast, first have some dried fruit soaked overnight in water or apple juice; it contains plenty of pectin and vitamins, and is just about the easiest food to digest.

Dr. Rudolph Ballantine, a physician who is an authority on Ayurvedic medicine, India's system of traditional medicine, which dates back at least several thousand years, takes another approach to fasting that you may find easier. To rejuvenate your digestive system on a regular basis, he recommends a *daily* fast about fourteen hours long. In other words, you might eat dinner at six in the evening, and then touch nothing until breakfast at eight the next morning. One reason this approach to fasting makes good physiological sense is that during the night, your bodily processes tend to slow down, so you need less fuel. Even if you don't fast in this fashion every day, you might try it once or twice a week.

Can Vitamins Be a Food Fallacy?

In 1988, Americans spent $3.1 billion on nutritional supplements, meaning nonprescription vitamins, minerals, and similar products. About 40 percent of the country pops nutritional supplements every day. All things considered, this is quite sensible. The average American's diet is not well balanced, and therefore is deficient in key nutrients, including vitamins A, C, B_2, B_6, folic acid, calcium, iron, and magnesium. And many people have habits that undermine good nutrition: they endure stress, they go on crash or fad diets, skip meals, rely on snacks. Or they take medications or indulge in cigarettes or alcohol, all of which can deplete your body's stores of nutrients. Especially for such people, supplements are a good idea.

Some vitamins fend off digestive trouble—vitamin D, for example, seems to help prevent colon cancer. And both vitamin A and zinc promote healing in cases of ulcers and colitis. But overdosing on certain vitamins can hurt your digestion. Don't feel that you're falling from Linus Pauling's good graces if indigestion obliges you to reduce your daily intake of vitamin C to a minimal 500 milligrams. Indeed, larger doses of vitamin C can cause uncomfortable gas and bloating. And taking megadoses of unnecessary iron, under the assumption that a little extra iron is good for everyone, not only can upset your digestion, but may undermine your health. One study found that men with high iron levels may be at a 40 percent greater risk for cancer.

The Virtues of Vegetables

Many mainstream nutrition experts consider vegetarianism a food fad at best—if not an outright food fallacy. I do not, and throughout history, many prominent thinkers have agreed. Playwright and philosopher George Bernard Shaw used to add the following postscript to all his letters: "Love animals; don't eat them!" And even the staid American Dietetic Association has opined that it may be easier for Americans to eat healthy diets if they switch to vegetarianism.

Sometimes patients who want to try vegetarianism ask me whether they will get enough protein, or enough vitamins and minerals. If you take up a vegetarian diet, you will have to be careful to eat balanced meals, especially if, besides meat and poultry, you also give up fish and animal products like milk, eggs, and cheese. Nutritionists at Baltimore's Vegetarian Resource Group have assembled a handy reference, a poster called "Vegetarianism in a Nutshell," which outlines how to change your diet and still eat sensibly (available from Vegetarians, P.O. Box 1463, Baltimore, Maryland 21203).

Think About It: How Do You Chew?

There have even been, and still are, fashionable ways of chewing your food. In the early 1900s, there was a fad for "Fletcherizing" your food, named for Horace Fletcher, who advocated chewing a mouthful at least forty times before swallowing. No doubt Fletcher's legacy to many small children was misery at the family dinner table!

Today, macrobiotics maven Michio Kushi goes beyond Fletcher: he admonishes his followers to chew *fifty* times before swallowing! I suspect, however, that Kushi simply wants to impress on you that a couple of chomps and a quick gulp simply aren't enough.

A 1989 Gallup poll found that only about one in three American adults eats at home and talks to others during meals, with no other distractions. Most—64 percent—read, worked, watched television, or did something else at the same time—and ate as quickly as possible.

Sensible weight-control programs often advise dieters to "watch how thin people eat." Often enough, those who have no trouble controlling their weight eat very slowly; they're only halfway through their first helping while everyone else is going for seconds. Eating slowly is essential to eating less—the slower you eat, the more likely you are to hear, and heed, your stomach's signals that say, "I'm full." Using chopsticks is helpful, but the easiest way to slow down is to start chewing every mouthful as thoroughly as possible. Your food will actually taste better; you may eat less, but you'll enjoy it more. Make a meal the sensory treat it is—not just an opportunity to shovel fuel down your gullet. Even Dr. Ehret, who wants you to give up "mucous food"—everything but fruit—believes in slow, careful chewing.

Thorough chewing is also the key to good digestion, which starts in your mouth. The more you chew each mouthful, the more thoroughly it will be drenched in saliva, which contains enzymes that begin breaking down your food even before you swallow it. The best way to make sure you chew properly is to eat when you're relaxed. One study at a dental school asked half of a group of students to do mental arithmetic while eating oat cereal, while the other half meditated. The meditators digested their cereal much more efficiently. Meditation promotes relaxation, which not only produces more saliva but also raises the levels of digestive enzymes in your saliva.

Think About It: How Do You Cope with Stress?

Note that I'm not asking, "Are you under stress?" As a modern American, I assume that you are. You may be familiar with a famous scale, published over twenty years ago, that rates forty-three events in terms of how stressful they are. Near the top are upsetting incidents that you might well expect to see on such a list, such as death of a spouse or close relative, divorce, being fired. But when you read through the list, you see numerous happenings that don't bring great loss but are cause for cheering: personal achievement, vacation, even Christmas. The point is, all these events involve change—and even pleasant, desirable change requires readjustment, and therefore stress. In today's world, change is a given, and so is stress.

Good nutrition is linked to fighting stress in a feedback loop, a concept from cybernetics in which a series of events are linked in such a way that you can't distinguish cause and effect. If you try to change one event, you change the whole system. That's how nutrition and stress are linked: nutrition affects how well you're able to cope with the physical and mental strains stress inflicts; poor nutrition puts even more stress on your body and mind; stress increases your need for nutrients.

Small wonder that stress can weaken your immune system, and has been implicated in life-threatening illnesses like heart disease and cancer. Researchers also estimate that stress plays a part in roughly 60 percent of gastrointestinal disorders, troubles that affect about 20 percent of American adults. Stress is often, though not always, a significant factor in flare-ups of ulcers, colitis, and irritable bowel syndrome. And it may cause nausea, diarrhea, indigestion and gas because under stressful circumstances, blood shifts away from the stomach. If you suffer from a chronic gastrointestinal problem, it's wise to take some preventive steps against the "stress epidemic."

How Stress Works

Some of my patients have trouble with the thought that stress might be contributing to their gastrointestinal problems. They insist that they have pains only when they're relaxing, and that any attempts they've made to stay calm didn't help their digestion. This isn't surprising in a society where staying "cool as a cucumber" and exhibiting "grace under pressure" are considered great virtues: if stress gives you a stomachache, how can you resemble Clint Eastwood?

It can be a relief to learn more about the way stress works, and its cumulative effect on the body; you won't feel as though you have to apologize because you "don't handle stress well." Stress may seem like a severe but temporary condition—a single event or situation. But stress can be considered a disease in itself, in which cumulative pressures have finally caused part of your body—namely, your gastrointestinal tract—to break down.

When you feel stress, your body senses a threat and mobilizes its resources in what is known as its "fight-or-flight" response to danger. As part of this complex physiological response, which evolved to keep prehistoric people out of the way of saber-toothed tigers, your adrenal glands release adrenaline, which helps pump extra glucose to your muscles in case you have to put up a fight or escape quickly. To ensure that you'll have as much energy available as possible, processes governed by your autonomic nervous system slow down. That means that blood courses away from your digestive tract to other muscles, and digestion slows. If you were hungry just before danger loomed, you lose your appetite.

Most modern difficulties—traffic jams or train delays that prevent us from arriving at work on time, crunching deadlines, strained relationships, and, of course, life's pleasant and unpleasant changes—aren't problems we can solve in physical ways: we can neither fight nor fly away from them. Dr. Herbert Benson, author of *The Relaxation Response*, whose groundbreaking research found that simple relaxation techniques reduce high blood pressure and risk of heart disease, has noted, "The 'fight-or-flight' response is no longer appropriate in the world we live in—can no longer meet today's social needs or stress."

Nevertheless, your body, once again behind the times, continues to mobilize against stress in prehistoric style. When this happens over and over again, as it does in modern life, your gastrointestinal system answers like the neighbors of the boy who cried wolf: it becomes less capable of responding effectively over and over again to false alarms. You have a fairly strong capacity to withstand an emergency—a massive dose of acute stress. However, recurring episodes that are lesser crises but add up to a way of life can do you in. If you take no precautions, months after a life-shaking loss or success your colitis may start troubling you.

Beware of the stress spiral: when you feel gastrointestinal symptoms coming on that may be due to stress, don't panic. You will only subject yourself to more stress as you berate yourself for not having whatever it takes to "handle" stress. You'll help yourself more by taking a positive attitude: by recognizing that you're under stress and your pains are a sign of a certain anatomical susceptibility. Just as some people eat more when they're under stress, and others lose their appetite, you simply happen, for various physiological reasons, to have your Achilles' heel located in your gut. Once you accept this, you can start thinking about taking appropriate action.

What Relaxation Techniques Can Do

What can you do to thwart your body's normal but outdated response to stress, so that your system doesn't turn on you and make you ill? After all, these responses are the work of your autonomic nervous system, which you think of as beyond your control. Well, medical science now acknowledges that what we used to term "psychosomatic" illness is real: your mind can affect your health in both a negative and a positive way. That means that you may have more control over autonomic processes than you think. You can learn to be flexible, to deal with life's tensions without turning them into stress that makes you ill.

If you've been following the Hoffman Program, you have already taken important steps to cut down stress by changing your diet. Researchers at Texas A & M University found that subjects who eliminated sugar and caffeine felt less stress, even if the rest of their diet remained the same. Smoking, alcohol, and seesaw dieting can add to stress. But if you're avoiding these bad habits, and still having gastrointestinal trouble, chances are you're leading a stressful life, or you wouldn't be experiencing symptoms. You can learn to relax, with the help of a number of relaxation techniques, including physical exercise, rhythmic breathing, practices where you move rhythmically as in yoga or the martial art of Tai Chi Chuan, meditation, muscle relaxation, visualization, biofeedback, or hypnotherapy.

Basically, all these techniques are gateways to autoregulation—control of your own bodily functions. From the first lesson you ever had in school on biology, you've learned that your nervous system has two arms, the voluntary and involuntary systems. When you decide to lift your right arm, that's the voluntary nervous system in action, sending signals from your brain to your arm muscles. When you digest, you don't think about it; your involuntary or autonomic nervous system simply goes to work.

But if you'd grown up in another culture—among Tibetan lamas, for example—you would have been taught that involuntary physiological processes can be brought under your conscious control. From your earliest years, you would have been trained to regulate your heart rate, your digestion, even your body's demand for oxygen. When a medicine man appears to heal a patient in a magic ritual, he is training the sick person to cure himself or herself. In fact, it's quite possible that we have a primitive self-healing response that our own culture teaches us to extinguish. After all, we grow up surrounded by images of illness and bodily dysfunction as environmental conditions that have overpowered us. Think of the countless times you've said, "It makes me sick" or "He gives me a pain." At the same time, you may have a hard time coming up with a common phrase that suggests taking control of a bodily process.

This, however, is what you are learning to do when you combat stress by taking up a relaxation program: you're starting to control your digestion.

Charting Your Own Stress

First of all, you have to figure out just how and when stress affects your digestion. Dr. Mark Schwartz of the Mayo Clinic has come up with an analogy that may help you understand stress's cumulative effect, and why it may be a hidden but very real contributor to your digestive difficulties. Think of yourself as a truck driver carrying several containers of various weights. Each container, which might represent your medical history, your weight, your eating habits, and so on, contributes differently to the "stress" on your truck as you start out rolling along every day. On a flat road, your truck travels well, but it may have trouble moving up hills.

Along the way, your truck has to pick up new containers—the sources of stress each day brings. The containers may represent your family, your job, the amount of sleep you get, and so on. To make room for these new containers on your truck, you have to choose which containers to set aside. Sometimes you may be able to empty part of a container. Or you may consider getting new shock absorbers to increase the truck's capacity.

Just as the truck's ability to travel smoothly depends on its day-to-day load of stress, your gastrointestinal symptoms may vary in the same way. If you suspect that stress is a part of your discomfort, try during this week to add some notes about stress to your food diary. Note any symptoms you have and their severity. You might place them on a scale ranging from very bad, to bad, medium, mild, none. If you do have symptoms, note any or all preceding stressful events: an argument with a friend or family member, bad news, extra work—or even a success of some kind. Keep up the diary as you start practicing stress control: every day, add whether you practiced.

I say "practice" because learning to relax is just like learning to play the piano, use a computer, ride a bike, speak Spanish, or any other skill. You learn only over time and only if you practice regularly. If you are faithful, however, your diary will tell you whether you are making progress: your symptoms will be much less frequent. I suggest you try simpler relaxation methods first, building up to some more complex ones. Not every technique works for everyone. But there's no need to feel obliged to experiment with all of them unless you're interested or want a change.

Find one or two that work consistently well for you. Then make relaxation practice a part of your daily life. Practicing is crucial, even when you feel fine. You'll be better prepared for days when digestive symptoms may strike. Having to do something every day for the sake of your health can be a daunting thought. But especially if you have a chronic problem, you need to maintain yourself, to stay in condition in case of stress. The cheering part is that stress management allows you to control your treatment yourself. You're in charge: you don't have to depend on your doctor or a bottle of medicine for relief—and you don't have to worry about side effects.

Physical Exercise

I suggest that you try exercise first—even though it may not be very easy right away if you're out of shape. Still, it's accessible and it's currently very fashionable. To stay fit and to combat stress, 23 million Americans jog, another 53 million walk, and 82 million ride bicycles weekly. Exercise relieves the physical and mental tension and the physiological changes that accompany stress. When your body mobilizes its resources but does not actually release "fight or flight" chemical messengers, feelings of physical and mental tension accumulate in your body, along with physiological stress products.

Vigorous exercise not only diverts your thoughts, it also rids your body of potentially harmful products like adrenaline. Production of adrenaline soars when you're nervous; continuous production can have adverse effects on bodily organs. Even modest amounts of exercise, like a brisk half-hour walk several times a week, seem to substantially reduce risk of colon cancer, probably because it increases bowel motility. Besides flushing out products that might wear out your body, exercise releases calming, beneficial ones like endorphins, which are natural opiates. When you're through exercising, you feel normally relaxed again. Don't think that you have to enroll in the toughest aerobics class available or pump iron like Arnold Schwarzenegger in order to benefit from exercise. Moderate forms like walking, golf, tennis, dancing, or daily stretching and warm-up exercises can do you just as much good, physically and mentally.

Remember that much as exercise helps, it is a source of stress in itself. When you exercise regularly, your body's needs for water, calories, certain minerals, and some vitamins increase. Water is particularly crucial: drink plenty during exercise, and afterward as well.

Although exercise generally aids digestion, it can do the opposite. For instance, if you have irritable bowel syndrome, running can cause spasms, forcing you to walk home. And near the finish line of a marathon, after several hours of intensive exercise, it's not unusual for runners to be afflicted with diarrhea. What's more, running for an hour or more can cause heartburn, even if you wait an hour or two after a meal to exercise. (Other forms of aerobic exercise don't seem to have the same effect on your esophagus.) Glaxo, the big British drug company that manufactures Zantac, an antiulcer drug that is one of the four best-selling drugs in the world, has been promoting its star product as preventing "runner's reflux." Rather than popping Zantac or taking an antacid tablet before a run, risking more digestive trouble, you may want to consider swimming for a change.

But some forms of exercise actually help digestive problems. One is a simple form of Dō-In, or Japanese self-massage based on the principles of acupuncture, an ancient system of Chinese medicine. Dō-In works because you stimulate points on the surface of your body, producing a balancing of the energy flow within a corresponding region or organ in your body. Properly performed, Dō-In can stimulate peristalsis. You simply massage your abdomen in a circular, clockwise direction, the same direction in which peristalsis moves through your gut.

Breathing and Meditation

The first thing a yoga course—or a singing coach, for that matter—teaches you is how to breathe from your diaphragm, a method of breathing more deeply and slowly. This type of breathing is the basis of breathing exercises for relaxation.

As you're breathing right now, I suspect that your abdomen doesn't move at all. But if you breathe from your diaphragm, you expand your lower abdomen and your rib cage—not just your chest. Your lower abdomen should balloon out when you inhale, and retract when you exhale. One yoga instructor suggests that when you are breathing, imagine that you are a glass filling with water, and then emptying: take about five seconds to breathe in, starting from your lower abdomen, then filling up through your lower rib cage to your chest. When you breathe out during the next five seconds, reverse this order: empty your chest first, then continue down, emptying your lower abdomen last.

Here's a simple yoga exercise that uses deep breathing to tone your digestive organs and promote circulation through your gut: every morning, as soon as you get out of bed, stand with your legs apart, lean forward, and place your hands midway down the tops of your thighs, fingers pointing inward. Standing in this position, breathe deeply in and out once. Then work your stomach muscles in and out as hard and as often as you can, until you need another breath. Repeat several times as a workout for your gastrointestinal tract before breakfast.

If you are quite flexible, there's another way to do this exercise. Kneel on the floor, then lie back flat, with shoulders on the floor and your legs folded up on either side of your body. Stretch your arms straight back over your head. Breathe in as deeply as possible; exhale and hold your breath as long as you can. Repeat several times. Those of you with back or knee problems, however, should consult your doctor or chiropractor before trying this.

Diaphragmatic breathing is essential for singers and for many athletes. It expands your lungs to capacity and ensures that you inhale plenty of oxygen to help your muscles work efficiently. Diaphragmatic breathing not only promotes deep breathing, it also slows breathing, so that you relax. Normally, you draw about 12 to 14 breaths a minute, although some people breathe as few as 5 or 6 times and others as often as 30 times a minute. When you breathe from the diaphragm, you aim for a steady rate of 9 to 12 breaths a minute, learning to control a function you had considered purely automatic.

Many forms of escape—a beer or glass of wine, an evening in front of television—seem to calm you, but don't promote deep physical relaxation. Concentrating on your breathing does. By emptying your mind so that all you think about is the quality of each breath—whether it is fast or slow, light or heavy, delicate or coarse, warm or cool—you clear your head and calm your body. Concentrated relaxation like this is a form of meditation. It lowers blood pressure, clears clogged arteries, and promotes healthy digestion.

You don't have to belong to a religion or have any deep interest in spirituality in order to practice and benefit from meditation. Since at least 200 B.C., it has been part of Eastern mysticism. Today, however, it is used alone as a means of relaxing—and healing.

There are many types of meditation, but all rely on concentration, contemplation, and mental repetition. It is easy to see how you can combine these qualities by deep, slow breathing. In Great Britain, the Western Buddhist Order, which has adapted the principles of Zen Buddhism for modern life, recommends a very practical, down-to-earth method of meditation: Count at the end of each outbreath; this helps to stop your mind from chattering away. Try to count up to ten outbreaths without distraction. But whenever you're distracted, which will be very often, especially when you first start meditating, go back to number one and start again. Concentrating on breathing is like listening to a musical note. Don't strain to hear it; just sit back.

When you feel you've mastered this first stage, move on to the second: counting before each inbreath. This requires a tiny bit more concentration. When you're ready for the third stage, stop counting; focus your whole awareness on each breath and its individual quality. In stage four, you concentrate on the point when you feel air coming in through your nostrils.

All this sounds simple, but it requires an almost athletic discipline. Meditation can be demanding exercise. Buddhists say there are five hindrances to meditation: pain; anxiety or restlessness; laziness; anger; and the "craving for sensuous experience," like wondering what's for lunch or having sexual fantasies. If you have a good deal of gastrointestinal trouble, pain may be your chief stumbling block. Consider that you're doing fine if you're able to practice for five or ten minutes a day, especially if you're a beginner.

Another useful form of meditation uses muscle relaxation techniques. These are becoming very popular; before major exams, you may see people around the room tensing every muscle as hard as they can for a few seconds—and then flopping back in their seats. The first step to using this method for concentrated relaxation is to run through your entire body, contracting each muscle in sequence for about seven seconds, and then letting go for about twice as long, before moving on to the next muscle. This exercise should take about twenty minutes.

The second stage of this form of meditation is to relax all your muscles without tensing them first. A good way to do this is to employ one of the many forms of visualization, or imagery, as a method of communicating with your autonomic nervous system. The use of imagery in healing dates back to Babylonia and Sumeria, survives in Oriental and tribal medical traditions, and is coming into vogue in Western medicine, especially for cancer patients. Scientific studies have confirmed that an image held in your mind can affect every single cell in your body.

To relax, for example, you can imagine that each muscle separately becomes heavy and warm. There are relaxation tapes that guide you through your entire body, focusing on each muscle and organ in turn, including your digestive organs. One tape asks you to imagine that each part of your body is progressively suffused with "warm, healing, golden light," until your whole being is inundated. Another method is to repeat a phrase like "calm" or "quiet" over and over as you relax each muscle. This is an especially good idea if you tend to wander off into daydreams, or start making lists of chores you think you ought to be doing instead of meditating.

Another form of visualization is to focus on your pulses in order to increase circulation—and thereby promote healing and better functioning—in various parts of your body, including your digestive organs. Assume a comfortable position in a quiet place where you can breathe deeply and start to relax. Concentrate on feeling the pulsation of your blood in your fingertips. Slowly transfer your concentration to pulsation in your arms, your shoulders, your neck, and so on, until you reach your lower abdomen or wherever you generally feel discomfort most often.

Once you have learned these techniques, you can carry them one step farther. Another type of meditation is to imagine yourself in a relaxing place. If you like the idea of bathing yourself in warm light, perhaps you prefer the thought of lying on a beach in Key West. Wherever you put yourself, make sure that your particular dream spot pleases all your senses. And make sure it is truly a spot where you feel relaxed; many people can't relax on a beach—the sun seems too strong, the wind and sand too gritty, and the surf too loud.

This kind of minimeditation is particularly useful in daily life. Once you master the technique, you can mentally whisk yourself away as soon as your dentist starts to drill, or whenever you know that if you're tense, the pain will be greater.

Homeopathy: A Little of What Ails You

Another way to combat stress is to take advantage of some alternative treatments for gastrointestinal ailments caused by stress. Chiropractic, homeopathy, and hypnotherapy are all legitimate medical disciplines that can help relieve stress in unorthodox ways. One of my patients who had been troubled with irritable bowel syndrome (IBS) for twenty years had reached the point of being "ready to try anything." She decided that a chiropractor might help her back pain, and perhaps the spasms that accompanied her IBS attacks as well.

Indeed, chiropractic treatments did provide temporary relief of her abdominal pain. This is not surprising: research done as early as 1921 found that slight spinal abnormalities could cause digestive disorders, including those of the esophagus, duodenum, and intestines. Many people with digestive diseases report a noticeable correlation between their back strains or pains and intestinal flare-ups. But like many other people who have consulted chiropractors, my patient discovered that a pleasant side benefit of the treatments was that they released muscle tension and stress, calming her considerably.

Homeopathy is another alternative healing system whose treatments can relieve stress. The fundamental principle behind all homeopathic treatments, known as the law of similars, is a basic principle of physics. Its application to healing dates back to the fourth century B.C. and Hippocrates, who said, "Through the like, disease is produced, and through the application of the like it is cured." This principle also underlies parts of Oriental, American Indian, and Indian, or Ayurvedic, medical traditions.

Instead of giving a sick person several different drugs, a homeopath prescribes a single medicine. Made from a vegetable, mineral, or animal substance, the medicine is meant to stimulate your body's immune system to help healing begin. The medicine is really a little bit of what ails you: a diluted, safe solution of a substance that in larger doses provokes the very symptoms you have. While modern pharmacists conclude that the larger the dose of a drug, the more powerful the effect, homeopaths take the opposite view: the smaller the dose, the stronger the effect.

Today, there are more than a thousand different homeopathic medicines listed in the *Homeopathic Pharmacopeia*. The FDA has exempted them from its rigorous testing procedures, on the grounds that,

HOMEOPATHY: A BRIEF HISTORY OF A SANE ALTERNATIVE

The father of homeopathy was Samuel Hahnemann (1755–1843), a respected German doctor who was opposed to bloodletting, massive doses of crude drugs, and other contemporary medical practices. He became intrigued by quinine, which comes from the bark of the cinchona tree and which relieves malaria. Hahnemann found that if he took quinine, he developed malarial symptoms. He deduced that symptoms were the first sign that your body is fighting an illness. If a medicine first made your symptoms worse, then it would make you better. By aggravating your symptoms, in other words, you could recover. This is how homeopathic remedies, all made from natural substances, work.

In the next two hundred years, homeopathy became very popular, and still is taught and widely practiced in Europe, including the Soviet Union, in parts of South America and Africa, as well as in India, Pakistan, and Sri Lanka. At the turn of the century, about 15 percent of American physicians considered themselves homeopaths. Charles Frederick Menninger, M.D., founder of the famous Menninger Clinic in Topeka, Kansas, was a homeopath. But after 1910, the opposition of the American Medical Association and major drug companies and the ascendance of hospital-based medicine resulted in a sharp decline in homeopathy in this country.

Today, although most Americans still know little or nothing about homeopathy, it has had a small renaissance beginning in the 1970s. In 1988, a French scientist, Jacques Benveniste, rocked the scientific world with an experiment that seemed to prove the efficacy of homeopathy. Although an investigating team from *Nature,* the prestigious British scientific journal, debunked Benveniste's experiment, teams in Italy, Israel, and Canada repeated it, and confirmed the Frenchman's results. For his part, Benveniste stands by his work, and warns, "There is more to come."

as an FDA spokesman said, "the dosages are so dilute that even cyanide would be safe. Traditional chemists would say that not even a molecule of the original substance is left." There is renewed interest in homeopathic medicines because they are incapable of inducing side effects, dependency, or iatrogenic disease. They are dispensed as tablets, drops, pills, powders, granules, and ointments, and it is possible to find doctors who are knowledgeable about homeopathic remedies. See the "Sources" section for addresses of homeopathic organizations.

There are some very effective homeopathic medications for stress-induced vomiting, diarrhea, and abdominal pain, which help reduce tension as well. For example, *Arsenicum album*, derived from arsenic, is poisonous in anything but a minute homeopathic dose. In that form, it relieves vomiting, diarrhea, and abdominal pain, and is especially effective in cases of food poisoning. Simultaneously, it relieves depression and anxiety. Another remedy for gastrointestinal distress and the stress at its root is *nux vomica*—which translates unappealingly as "the vomit nut." It relieves heartburn, nausea, diarrhea, gas, and bloating.

Biofeedback: Watching Your Body Work

Biofeedback is shorthand for external psychophysiological feedback. Basically, this relaxation technique uses electronic instruments to provide you with information, in the form of measurements and visual and auditory signals, about what is going on inside your body. If you use biofeedback in conjunction with visualization, your imaging will tell your autonomic nervous system what to do, and the instrumentation will tell you how well it carried out your instructions.

To use biofeedback, you need a trained professional's help. Your trainer attaches electrodes or electronic transducers to parts of your body to send signals to equipment that reads your heart rate, blood pressure, hand temperature, muscle tension, galvanic skin response, or brain activity. The Menninger Foundation, which has studied a Hindu yogi to confirm his impressive control over his heart rate, brain waves, and other autonomic functions, has successfully pioneered the use of biofeedback as a drug-free means of lowering blood pressure. But it remains unclear how effective biofeedback really is as a way of reducing stress, although some studies have indicated that it is useful. In 1988 the U.S. Army commissioned a surprising study. It found that biofeedback training relaxed muscles and produced brainwaves suggesting a calm state of mind, but had little significant effect on stress.

Nevertheless, biofeedback has been used to help treat irritable bowel syndrome, fecal incontinence, vomiting, ulcers, and esophageal disorders. The goal of biofeedback training for gastrointestinal troubles is to teach you to recognize stress symptoms that often accompany the onset of your pain. As you learn to decrease your physiological response to stress, you often are able to decrease the intensity and duration of gastrointestinal symptoms. I believe that biofeedback is useful because it provides you with two essential ingredients of stress control: feedback, which is key to learning any skill, even the knack of relaxing, and opportunities to practice.

For example, the most useful measurements in treating abdominal pain are your hand temperature and your muscle activity. Changing the temperature of your hands or releasing muscular tension seems to relieve gastrointestinal symptoms. If you relax by focusing your attention on exactly how your hands are feeling, and then imagine that they are warm, they may begin to warm slightly. But to be sure of what is happening, so you can learn to make this happen whenever you need to relax, you need feedback. Biofeedback will give you objective information.

According to Steven L. Fahrion, Ph.D., of the Menninger Foundation Voluntary Controls Program, you can begin to learn to control stress with biofeedback training in about a half hour. Your trainer will place a sensor on, among other spots, the little finger of your left hand. Perhaps because of brain dominance, this finger's temperature is always the first and the fastest to warm or cool. Then your trainer will suggest that you make a conscious attempt to relax, repeating to yourself a phrase like, "My hands are warm and heavy," as you try to imagine exactly what that feels like. Or you can imagine that you're warming your hands over an open fire, that you're sunning them or dipping them in warm water, or that you've just put on fleece-lined mittens. Above all, Dr. Fahrion says, your trainer will emphasize that you're *letting* your hands warm, not *making* them: "If you simply trust your body to do what you're asking it to do, then you'll find that it will."

Meanwhile, other electrodes on your forehead will measure your muscle activity. Dr. Fahrion says that, in about 65 percent of patients, muscle tension changes with hand temperature, relaxing when their hands warm. While stress decreases the flow of blood to your gastrointestinal tract, relaxation promotes circulation and, therefore, better digestion. Once biofeedback has told you that your relaxation techniques have definite, positive, physiological results, you can put them to use whenever stress threatens to overwhelm you. By warming your hands, you calm your emotions and relax your muscles, thus quieting your body and settling your stomach.

Self-Hypnosis: Settling Your Stomach Through Trances

Many gastrointestinal disorders, including ulcers, ulcerative colitis, diverticulitis, irritable bowel syndrome, diarrhea, and constipation, are heavily tied to your personal response to stress. If you are in emotional distress, you may be in gastrointestinal distress as well. In fact, for some people, gastrointestinal upset is their only sign of depression or anxiety. Such people are not consciously aware of their emotions, but their guts are!

According to Gérard Sunnen, a psychiatrist who specializes in hypnotherapy, people emerging from their first trance frequently exclaim, "I never felt so relaxed before!" Hypnotherapy and self-hypnosis can promote healing and control excessive anxiety that exacerbates gastrointestinal upset. Sunnen has used hypnotherapy to successfully treat ulcers and ulcerative colitis, and some new studies have confirmed that hypnotherapy can help improve severe cases of irritable bowel syndrome, and also prevent relapses in 50 percent of patients with chronic duodenal ulcers.

Exactly how the sleeplike condition of a hypnotic trance works to promote relaxation, suppress pain, and foster healing is not clear, but the American Medical Association endorsed hypnotherapy as a means of pain control more than thirty years ago. Like biofeedback, self-hypnosis is a technique you must learn from a professional. Dr. Sunnen says that one or two hour-long sessions will tell you if this relaxation technique is right for you. Then you'll need four or five more sessions to learn how to put yourself in a trance state, which is really a state of profound relaxation.

The idea of "being hypnotized" panics some people; they associate it with being under the control of some Svengali. Actually, Dr. Sunnen says, in self-hypnosis, which he calls "a talent that can be learned," you choose the direction, depth, and even the length of your own trance. You decide whether you will emerge after a certain time limit or will lapse into sleep—an option that insomniacs often choose. As you put yourself into a trance state, you guide yourself to a new state of mind, thus reducing stress and strengthening your immune system. While in a trance state, you allow yourself to experience what tension or a particular gastrointestinal symptom feels like. Then you let it go, and in doing so, you are able to dispel it.

To guide you into a trance state, a hypnotherapy professional may use the classic swinging coin, or ask you to focus on an image like a mandala, to still your conscious, analytical mind. Or you may use visualization, imagining, for example, that "My body feels warm and heavy" or "I feel very light all over." Your guide will help you define the state you're looking for: you feel relaxed, but alert; your thoughts are irrelevant; you are becoming more and more keenly aware of your body. Then your guide may suggest that you meditate for a while on your body's energies.

At this point, you're ready to employ some healing techniques. Your guide might suggest that you create a waking dream that might trigger memories or illuminate some reasons why you may use gastrointestinal symptoms to express anxiety. Or you may learn to use your increased awareness of your physical being to become more cognizant of your internal organs. You might focus on what your symptoms feel like, and then conjure images that will soothe or neutralize them. For example, you might concentrate on the burning sensation of your ulcer, and then think of cooling it with falling snow, a waterfall, gentle rainfall. Later, you can recall these healing images whenever your pain returns.

Finally, recent studies have found that hypnosis can suppress your perception of pain, explaining why some hypnotized patients can undergo surgery without anesthesia. While in your trance, you can create a symptom—actually bring on a sensation you dread—and then banish it. By creating it and then letting it go, you extend your range of control over your autonomic nervous system. You systematically train yourself to be less sensitive to pain.

Dr. Sunnen reports that hypnotherapy further promotes relaxation because it helps you meditate by enhancing your ability to create mental images. And while meditation can take four to six weeks of daily practice to begin to master, you experience the benefits of self-hypnosis in less time. Dr. Sunnen recommends daily practice—or, at the very least, every other day. For the first two weeks, take daily notes to keep track of your progress and any difficulties you have, so that your hypnotherapist can help you.

One Last Word Before You Relax . . .

A new study has found that a good self-help book may be enough to help you relax. The title that clinical psychologists recommend most often to anxious patients is Dr. Herbert Benson's *The Relaxation Response*. But perhaps just reading this chapter alone has soothed you. How does your gut feel now?

When You Need More Help

If you're plagued with a chronic gastrointestinal problem that no gastroenterologist seems able to fix and that the Hoffman Seven-Week Program has not alleviated, don't despair. There are new, effective and, for the most part, simple self-treatments available for most of those minor miseries that aren't dangerous, but certainly are uncomfortable, sometimes embarrassing, and occasionally disabling. And there are also new ways to treat serious, life-threatening illnesses like ulcers or colitis. Just as the Hoffman Program uses diet to prevent everyday gastrointestinal distress, you can change your eating habits in ways that will help stave off major problems like gallstones and intestinal cancer.

CHAPTER · 8

New Treatments
for Chronic Miseries

*"My wind exploded like a thunder-clap.
. . . Iaso blushed a rosy red
And Panacea turned away her head
Holding her nose: my wind's not frankincense."*

—Aristophanes, Plutus

Gas and Belching

Let's start with those gastric *faux pas* that Aristophanes played for
laughs. Americans consider belching a social misdemeanor, but in
some parts of the world, a loud burp after a hearty meal is a compli-
ment to the chef and a tribute to your host. Chaucer, Rabelais, and
Joyce delighted in burps and farts; Chaucer actually invented the word
"fart." Fraternity boys relish "lighting farts." Other people leave the
house when they sense that they have to pass gas, or keep matches
near the toilet to cover the smell of the gas that accompanies a bowel
movement. Television ads, especially the ones you see on Thanksgiv-
ing afternoon, give the impression that intestinal gas can be conquered
with over-the-counter remedies.

This is simply not true. Smelly and embarrassing as flatus can be,
you have no choice. All of us have gas, a natural by-product of digestion, in our gastrointestinal tract, and must get rid of it somehow.

Even Hippocrates, who heard so many complaints about gas that he wrote an essay on the problem called "The Winds," acknowledged that "Passing gas is necessary to well-being." On a normal day, you take care of your well-being by means of approximately 15 belches or farts, passing roughly 40 milliliters of gas (about one ounce) per emission. In short, there is no cure for "breaking wind," nor should there be.

But too much gas may be a sign that something is wrong. Perhaps you are suffering from a food intolerance or irritable bowel syndrome. Excess gas also may signal a serious problem, like an ulcer or an abdominal obstruction. And too much of a certain ingredient of intestinal gas, methane, may indicate an improper balance in your intestinal flora.

WHERE GAS COMES FROM, WHERE IT GOES

The gas you release in belching comes from the upper portion of your gastrointestinal tract. It got there because you swallowed it as you talked, ate, or drank. The faster you do those things, the more air you swallow. As much as 70 percent of intestinal gas comes from swallowed air. You may be taking in even more air by smoking, sipping through a straw, drinking carbonated or foaming beverages, eating dishes made with beaten eggs or whipped cream, chewing gum or sucking candies, or even wearing loose dentures.

I've mentioned earlier that eating slowly and chewing thoroughly are watchwords for improving your digestion. Rabelais describes a queen who took this idea very seriously: she hired masticators to chew her food for her! You don't have to go this far, but careful chewing is especially helpful if you want to belch less often. Effervescent over-the-counter remedies, like Alka-Seltzer, are no help to belchers. Like carbonated beverages, these remedies make you belch even more. You may feel that your problem is being solved because you're allowing gas to escape as you're belching. In reality, your medication is triggering extra belching because you're swallowing more air along with your remedy. The more air you swallow, the more distention you may feel in your esophagus and stomach, and the more you may belch. Sometimes reflux and heartburn accompany belching.

Although you release most air you swallow in belching, some passes down your gut and out your rectum in flatulence. Some of the gas you release this way is made in your lower intestine, when bacteria ferment undigested food. As some researchers have observed, "In champagne, fermentation produces bubbles; in the large intestine—flatus."

Intestinal gas actually is a combination of several gases, including nitrogen—by far the largest component, sometimes as much as 90 percent—and oxygen, which, like nitrogen, comes from swallowed air. Carbon dioxide, hydrogen, and methane, better known as swamp gas, all result from the normal workings of your intestinal flora, along with a few molecules of butyric acid and trace substances with resonant names like putrescine and cadaverine. A little of these goes a long way, contributing heavily to flatulence's distinctive fragrance. I can attest to butyric acid's staying power: I was an undergraduate at Columbia University during the 1969 student riots. Someone pinched a small vial of butyric acid from the chemistry lab and hurled it inside the lobby of a campus building. This homemade stink bomb was incredibly effective: for months afterward, whenever I hurried through that lobby on my way to class, a stench hung in the air!

WHAT GAS MAY MEAN

If you feel bloated and your waistline is visibly distended after meals, you may have only a normal amount of gas—you just can't handle it properly. One possible explanation is poor tone in your abdominal muscles: fifty crunches (sit-ups in which you elevate your head and chest only) a day, or even the yoga exercises I described in the previous chapter, may make a big difference. Another possible cause is irritable bowel syndrome, a minor but uncomfortable problem which I discuss in detail later in this chapter.

If you suffer from irritable bowel syndrome, you probably have only an average amount of gas, but because of your particular nervous system, you feel as though you have too much. You don't really have excess gas; it's just that a normal amount makes you feel pain and distention.

Some other causes of gassy discomfort may mimic irritable bowel syndrome, but turn out to be much less complex. Gas can decrease markedly if you make some changes in your diet. You may feel better if you avoid certain foods or eat smaller servings of others.

• *Lactose Intolerance:* Except for people of northern European descent, many adults can't digest milk and its products well. Even if you have no trouble with dairy foods now, you may become less tolerant as you grow older. If you suspect that lactose intolerance is the cause of your gas, ask your doctor for a test that measures the amount of hydrogen in your breath. A certain amount is a clear sign of lactose intolerance.

However, a hydrogen breath test does require expensive, sophisticated equipment that your doctor may not have on hand. Instead, you can ask for a variation on the glucose tolerance test. Your doctor draws a blood sample and measures your blood sugar. Then you swallow a beverage containing lactose. One hour and again two hours later, your doctor tests your blood sugar again. If it has not gone up, you have not absorbed any of the lactose you drank—clear evidence that you cannot break lactose down into absorbable sugars.

Once you stop eating dairy products, except for fermented ones like yogurt, your gas trouble should clear up. Taking lactase supplements or eating yogurt (the yogurt culture has already digested lactose for you) also will settle your digestion.

• **Sorbitol Intolerance:** Do you have more gas now that you've gone on a diet? Perhaps you're unable to tolerate sweeteners like sorbitol or its relative, xylitol. Sorbitol is a natural substance, but like some other artificial sweeteners, it is a carbohydrate that your small intestine does not absorb. Instead, sorbitol arrives intact in your lower intestine, where bacteria ferment it, resulting in extra gas.

Sorbitol is a common ingredient in "sugarless" or "dietetic" foods like sugarless gum or diet margarine. If you're sensitive to sorbitol and have ingested quite a bit because you're trying to lose weight, you may have diarrhea. Even some fruits, especially cherries and plums, are high in sorbitol. Fruit can also cause gas if you're sensitive to fructose.

An elimination diet or a hydrogen breath test is the best way to find out whether your gas trouble is definitely due to sorbitol intolerance. If you cannot tolerate sorbitol, try avoiding dietetic foods and lose weight by sticking to low-fat foods and passing up sweets.

• **Candida's Fertilizers:** Excess gas may be a symptom of a *Candida* infection. *Candida* turns your gut into a factory that processes carbohydrates into alcohol, carbon dioxide, and various by-products. Just as dough needs a sugar "starter" to rise, *Candida* is helped along considerably if you eat sugar on top of carbohydrates. And just as yeast forms air pockets in rising dough, *Candida* adds more air to your intestinal tract. If you suspect that *Candida* is what is making your insides rumble, avoid sugary foods and ask a doctor who is knowledge-able about nutrition for a *Candida* test.

• ***Newfound Fiber:*** It's a cruel fact: some foods give you gas because they are good for you. They contain fiber which, just like sorbitol, is fermented by your colonic bacteria. The ability to digest fiber comfortably is quite individual. You may have trouble with a bowl of high-fiber cereal that someone else downs quite happily. Although a high-fiber diet can eliminate constipation and help you lose weight, it can cause an uncomfortable amount of gas.

In the early days of the space program, the U.S. Department of Agriculture developed a system for measuring the "flatus-producing effect" of different foods—key information for astronauts who have to orbit for days and days in a small space capsule! Certain high-fiber foods seem to cause more gas than others. Among them are beans, celery, broccoli, cauliflower, carrots, onions ("good for the heart but they make you fart," as the saying goes), cabbage, apples, and raisins. I've also noticed that my patients sometimes report trouble with some foods containing oligosaccharides, or complex sugars, that resist diges-tion. Such foods include artichokes, barley, Brussels sprouts, coconut meat, figs, honey, kohlrabi, molasses, mulberries, nuts, rye seeds, soybeans, wheat, and yeast.

If you're trying to eat more fiber, it's a good idea to introduce fibrous foods into your diet slowly, in small amounts. Generally speak-ing, your gut adjusts best if it's allowed to adjust slowly. You certainly should not shy away from high-fiber foods, because in order to reduce gas, you have to avoid constipation. If you are constipated, the passage of food through your gastrointestinal tract slows down, stepping up fermentation. So do eat high-fiber foods and drink plenty of water.

HOW TO HANDLE BEANS

Especially if you are on a vegetarian diet, you are likely to turn to beans as a major source of protein. A cup of cooked beans provides a quarter of your daily protein requirement—with almost no fat. What's more, beans are rich in iron, folic acid, and calcium, and help lower your cholesterol almost as much as oats do.

Unfortunately, beans, like seeds, contain substances that prevent your intestinal tract from completely absorbing them. When you first start eating beans regularly, you are likely to be bothered by gas. After a while, your gut usually adjusts, and your gas diminishes. Some beans do produce more gas than others: soy, black, and pink beans are heavyweights; green, pinto, and small white beans are middleweights: and black-eyed peas, lima and garbanzo beans are welterweights.

You can also cut down on flatulence by as much as 60 percent if you try a special technique for cooking dried beans. Soak the beans in water for four or five hours, and then discard the water. Add fresh water, cook the beans for half an hour, and then discard the water again. If you need to cook the beans any longer, add more water, cook them, and then discard this water as well. This cooking method does have a drawback: some bean protein and water-soluble B vitamins will be lost. But enough nutrients remain to make eating beans well worth your while.

You can also reduce gas by cooking beans in your usual manner and adding kombu, a sea vegetable that is popular in Japanese cuisine and available in health-food stores. When the beans are ready, discard the kombu along with the cooking water. Kombu reduces flatulence without affecting the beans' nutritional content.

A method of reducing gas that actually enhances vitamin content is to sprout beans and seeds. You can do this at home, even in the dead of winter. Simply place any kind of beans or seeds in a wide-mouthed jar and soak them in water. Cover the jar with nylon mesh or cheese-cloth and let the jar stand overnight. Discard the water the next morning, and rinse the beans with fresh water. Store the jar in a warm, dark place for the next two to four days, rinsing the beans twice daily. You may prefer to use a commercial sprouter, for sale in kitchen-supply and some health-food stores. Use the sprouted beans in salads. Sprouting beans makes them easier to digest, even when you eat them raw.

PREVENTING GAS: REACH FOR CHARCOAL

Most over-the-counter and prescription remedies for gas, like Di-Gel, contain simethicone, an agent that reduces the surface tension of gas bubbles so that large ones break into smaller ones and burst more easily. Although this ingredient sounds quite effective, most tests have found that while simethicone works well for gas in the small intestine and reduces belching, it is no better for treating gas in the lower intestine and flatulence than placebos.

On the other hand, activated charcoal, a substance that binds a variety of chemicals, does seem to work well for both kinds of gas.

Possibly charcoal binds either gas itself or the substances in your food that produce it. While activated charcoal is not absorbed into your body from your intestine, charcoal does tend to bind any vitamins or drugs, including birth-control pills, that you may be taking and prevent them from being absorbed. If you need supplements or medication, charcoal is not an alternative for you. Otherwise, take two tablets before a meal rich in gas-producing dishes, and another two afterward.

THE HOFFMAN ANTI-GAS DIET

For patients who are particularly troubled by gas, I have combined the best ways of fighting excess gas into a special antigas regimen:

• Take a tip from food-combining enthusiasts: eat fruit and drink fruit juices only a half hour before or two hours after a meal, to reduce fermentation as much as possible.

• Chew all your food as slowly and thoroughly as possible. If you gulp down your meals, you swallow your food in lumps, which are harder to digest and remain longer in your small intestine, where their residue may ferment.

• Paradoxically, both diarrhea and constipation can exacerbate gas. Some vitamins and supplements also can cause gas. Vitamin C can be particularly gas-forming. Reduce your dosage to about 500 milligrams a day. Supplements can be troublesome, too: iron can upset your stomach, and magnesium can give you diarrhea and consequently gas. Go on a mini-elimination diet: stop taking all your vitamins, and then add them back one by one every day. If there is a vitamin culprit, you will find it.

• If you are taking calcium supplements, consider whether you should change the type you use. Tums are a popular choice as a supplement because they contain calcium carbonate. But calcium carbonate can cause gas and constipation because of its chalky consistency. Another popular source of calcium is dolomite supplements, named for the Dolomite Mountains in Yugoslavia. To prevent a similar hardening of whatever is passing through your intestinal tract, switch to calcium citrate, which is not binding and won't give you gas.

• If you eat beans, follow my suggestions for cooking them or sprout them first.

• Instead of Di-Gel, try Phazyme 95, an over-the-counter medication that contains the highest dose of simethicone available in a single tablet.

A BRIEF HISTORY OF HERBAL MEDICINE

The use of herbs to heal probably dates back to prehistory. Folk medicine and ancient medical traditions, such as Chinese medicine and Ayurvedic medicine, India's system of traditional medicine, rely heavily on herbal remedies. Today, some of our best known and most useful drugs, such as digitalis for the heart, were developed from plants. The Indian government is underwriting research into the healing potential of Ayurvedic herbs, and one major American drug company, Merck, is collaborating with the University of Beijing on a study of the medicinal potential of over forty drugs commonly used in traditional Chinese medicine. The National Academy of Science has concluded that nearly half of Chinese medicinal herbs are scientifically valid.

The great advantage of herbal remedies is that they are much less likely than drugs to have side effects. After all, plants have been part of our environment for millions of years, and so our bodies have evolved the ability to tolerate and benefit from them. Herbal teas have therapeutic effects, but most herbal medicines are prescribed in the form of tinctures, made by chopping some of the plant's leaves, roots, and flowers, and immersing them in a solution of alcohol and water. Alcohol extracts the plant's healing compounds, and preserves them as well.

Some herbs are also available in tablet or capsule form. One is garlic, among the most versatile and effective of all natural remedies. Researchers are investigating its ability to lower cholesterol and blood pressure. Garlic also fights parasites, stimulates digestion, and inhibits the growth of harmful species of intestinal bacteria. Another herb, wormwood, also known as artemisia, is a good antidote for parasites.

Surprisingly, some hot, tonic, or aromatic bitter herbs can soothe an upset stomach. For indigestion or sour upset stomach, I recommend a hot bitter, raw ginger, which can also relieve seasickness. I also like a stomach tonic made up by Daniel Gagnon, a Santa Fe, New Mexico, herbalist, of several bitter herbs, including catnip, fennel, lavender, star anise, cayenne, cardamom, angelica, gentian, and prickly ash berries. For sluggish digestion and stasis, I use a digestive tonic composed of gentian,

(continued from opposite page)

quassia, angelica, goldenseal, bayberry, and cardamom. Ayurvedic physicians rely on black pepper, mustard, and fenugreek to intensify salivation and stimulate your stomach. Chamomile, peppermint, or raspberry leaf tea can ease cramps and morning sickness. Meadowsweet can soothe damaged gastric mucosa and reduce stomach acidity, and help relieve heartburn. James A. Duke, Ph.D., the U.S. Department of Agriculture's expert on herbs, reports that for years, his wife has relied on cinnamon toast for gastric upset.

If herbal medicine is so helpful and safe, why isn't there more research into it, and why isn't it widely promoted? One reason is that a drug company has to spend about $125 million on studies and research to prove that a new drug is safe and effective before marketing it. Since it is very difficult to patent an herb, no company wants to invest in a new medicine to which it would not have exclusive rights, and for which it might not be able to recover its research costs. At present, the herbal medicine industry is proposing legislative reforms to ease the FDA's approval process for herbs like peppermint, a remedy for irritable bowel syndrome. Hence, the reformers say, these herbs ought to be "grandfathered" into popular medical practice.

• Add milk-free acidophilus supplements and herbal tonics to your meals. I give my patients Ileocecal Tonic, which contains quassia, bistort, ginger, angelica, and bayberry. According to James A. Duke, a botanist who is the U.S. Department of Agriculture's authority on herbs, folk medicine credits both epazote and sweet annie with the ability to reduce flatus. Other herbs that soothe your intestinal tract and reduce gas include cumin, coriander, peppermint (which you can take in the form of peppermint oil supplements or peppermint tea), turmeric, anise (which tastes like licorice), and fenugreek, which tastes a little like maple syrup and was the main ingredient in Lydia Pinkham's Vegetable Compound, the famous turn-of-the-century cure-all.

Hiccups

Hiccups are not caused by gas, but by intermittent involuntary spasms of your diaphragm. Researchers speculate that these spasms occur if your swallowing reflex and the movement of your diaphragm as you breathe are not coordinated. Eating too fast can certainly trigger this kind of disharmony. If you gobble, you shove food down your esophagus and through your diaphragm too rapidly, overloading your autonomic nervous system's circuits and causing spasmodic contractions that erupt as hiccups.

Because hiccups are a sign that your central nervous system is disrupted, amitriptyline, a common antidepressant, is sometimes prescribed to treat them—without notable success. Many of the old formulas you probably heard as a child—slow sips of water, sucking on a sugar cube—are more effective than drugs. Even Mary Poppins's formula, a spoonful of dry white granulated sugar, makes your hiccups subside. When sugar fails, folk remedies include a jigger of vinegar and chewing on a lemon wedge saturated with bitters.

Granulated substances like sugar, as well as any action that controls your breathing or swallowing, probably work because they send your diaphragm a clear signal that can unscramble your spasms and banish your hiccups. Biotin, a B vitamin, also seems to ease hiccups. Since biotin deficiency can cause neurological disorders, perhaps biotin has a powerful effect on your brain and nervous system, and can override the crossed signals that cause hiccups.

Heartburn

I've mentioned that chronic halitosis can be an early sign of a lack of hydrochloric acid or of a bacterial infection that can lead to an ulcer. But unless your bad breath is due to sinus trouble, tooth decay, or gum disease—and you should certainly have both medical and dental checkups to rule out these possibilities—it can also be a sign of heartburn.

Up to 10 percent of all Americans have heartburn every day; at least one third of the country feels the occasional twinge, and this complaint is very common during pregnancy. Though some expectant mothers find that heartburn can be quite disabling, it usually vanishes after the baby is born. Heartburn usually feels like a burning pain in your chest—it can even be mistaken for a heart attack. Sometimes you can taste the acid reflux that causes your pain: you feel your food coming back toward your mouth, with an acidic or bitter taste. Most often, you feel the pain of heartburn after meals or when you lie down in bed. Although severe heartburn can indicate dangerous esophageal disease, it is rarely little more than an annoyance.

When you feel the burning sensation of heartburn, the contents of your stomach, known as acid reflux, are washing back up your esophagus toward your mouth. If the reflux is heavy enough, it can irritate or inflame your esophagus—which is probably the cause of most of your discomfort. Normally, the point where your stomach joins your esophagus is kept closed by a muscle called the lower esophageal sphincter. When you swallow, this sphincter relaxes so that food can pass into your stomach, but then it quickly closes.

However, several factors can loosen your lower esophageal sphincter so that it does not close promptly or completely. One of them is an aging gut: according to Dr. Donald O. Castell, who has studied esophageal disease and heartburn, "Most of us who have heartburn don't remember having it as teenagers." Heartburn during pregnancy usually starts during the first trimester, when hormones relax uterine muscles to accommodate the growing fetus. Unfortunately, these hormones affect your lower esophageal sphincter as well.

This kind of heartburn can't be avoided, but you can prevent other forms. Smoking and being overweight can exacerbate heartburn, which often disappears once you quit smoking or lose weight. Particular foods, especially fried and fatty foods, alcohol, tomatoes, citrus fruits, coffee, and chocolate, seem to irritate your esophageal lining or relax your sphincter muscle, and trigger reflux and heartburn. A few afterdinner drinks tend to bring on nighttime reflux. Besides eliminating troublesome foods and drink, you can enlist gravity's help: place the head of your bed on six-inch blocks. This seems to reduce heartburn by minimizing the flow of reflux from your stomach into your esophagus at night.

A recent study found that running seems to cause "runner's reflux" and consequently heartburn. Other forms of exercise in which you jostle your body less—bicycling, for example, or working out with weights—don't seem to have the same effect, unless you exercise right after a meal. Dr. Castell speculates that while running, you swallow a fair amount of air resulting in the desire to belch. As you do so, some of the acid jostling in your stomach sneaks back up your esophagus.

When you consult a conventional doctor about heartburn, he or she may recommend that you swallow barium and then have your upper gastrointestinal tract x-rayed. Then you may hear, "Aha! No wonder you have heartburn. You have a hiatal hernia." Before your esophagus joins your stomach, it passes through an hourglass-shaped opening, or hiatus, in the wall of your diaphragm. This is the point at which your lower esophageal sphincter opens and then closes to keep acid in your stomach. A hernia means that one of your organs is protruding through the wall of the cavity which surrounds it. So when you have a hiatal hernia, part of your stomach is pocketing out through the hiatus in your diaphragm.

The trouble is, this painless condition is so common that its diagnosis is almost meaningless. It can occur in anyone, even newborns; according to some estimates, 50 percent of patients over 50 have hiatal hernias. Only about 5 percent of cases ever require surgery. Chiropractic care can help restore your diaphragm's muscular strength, and some changes in your diet and habits can clear up heartburn. Avoid lying down after meals or eating large meals at night, especially right before you go to bed.

Studies show that doctors' most popular remedy for heartburn, regular doses of acid-suppressing drugs, notably Tagamet and Zantac, are effective in treating reflux. (Nevertheless, for the most part, these drugs are little help for ordinary dyspepsia, or "sour stomach.") Aloe vera and bismuth, the active ingredient in Pepto-Bismol, are quite helpful for reflux. My ulcer diet (see next chapter) can relieve heartburn as well.

Many cases clear up if you acidify your stomach by taking supplemental hydrochloric acid. I've always thought that this was one of the most remarkable phenomena in medicine—that a condition that's almost always treated with antacids can be reversed by administering acid. However, this approach really does make physiological sense. If your stomach does not produce enough hydrochloric acid, you can really feel as though food is "stuck in your craw."

Constipation

Most conventional doctors define constipation as the inability to have a bowel movement after three days or more—and as I've noted already, I believe that much more frequent bowel movements are a boon to health. Hippocrates himself held that, for optimal health, you should defecate "twice or thrice" daily. When feces remain in your colon too long, they become hard, dry, and difficult to expel; in short, you become constipated. The more time passes between bowel movements, the more likely you are to have hard stools and pain or even bleeding during elimination. Constipation is so common in Western countries that most doctors dismiss it as unworthy of medical attention. The main cause of constipation, I am convinced, is the American way of life: too much fat and sugar, not enough fiber and exercise. Too much alcohol, coffee, and tea—Americans' favorite drinks—also may bring on constipation by depleting your body of fluids. Forty million Americans take laxatives—eight million of us habitually. Laxatives account for 1 percent of all doctors' prescriptions, and we spend more than $250 million every year on nonprescription laxatives—over 700 different products—in search of a cure for constipation.

There are several different kinds of laxative. Stimulant or irritant laxatives cause rhythmic contractions in your small or large intestine; osmotic laxatives, such as milk of magnesia, cause water to secrete into your colon; stool softeners, such as docusate sodium, moisten your stool and prevent it from becoming too hard and dry; bulk agents, such as Metamucil, hold water and make your stool softer and easier to pass; lubricants, such as mineral oil, also soften your stool and allow it to slip through your colon more easily. But laxatives are usually unnecessary and can be dangerous. If you use them heavily, they can give you diarrhea. With the exception of bulk agents, any laxative can become habit-forming: your body's natural mechanism starts to rely on laxatives to prompt bowel movements, and can't work without them. Routine use of the most common ingredient in irritant laxatives, castor oil, damages the lining of your intestinal tract. Too much of another popular laxative, mineral oil, can interfere with your ability to absorb certain vitamins and minerals. And paradoxically, unless you drink plenty of water when you use bulk laxatives, they can make your constipation worse. Elvis Presley's private physician once told an interviewer that his patient suffered from chronic constipation, and added, "I felt it probably related to a long history of laxative abuse."

Although constipation can make you feel bloated, heavy, and uncomfortable, it is not an illness. Rather, it is a symptom that something is wrong with your diet or your habits, or even that you are going through an emotional change. But it can signal a problem like irritable bowel syndrome or a serious hidden disorder, such as colon cancer. Women, thanks to anatomical differences, tend to have a weak pelvic floor, and therefore seem to be more susceptible to constipation than men. Sometimes, hormonal activity is to blame; constipation is very common during pregnancy.

Older people are five times more likely to complain of constipation. Lack of exercise and the natural slowing of the aging gut play a part here. Older people also take more prescription drugs, some of which, such as antidepressants and pain-killers, can be constipating. So can some over-the-counter remedies, such as iron supplements and antacids that contain aluminum. But for many older people, the real trouble is that they have relied on laxatives all their lives, and now their bad habits are coming home to roost.

Sometimes patients tell me that they become constipated whenever they're away from home, even for an overnight stay. They tell me, "It must be the water." Actually, the reason is simply a shift in your routine; a change of place and habits, even for just twenty-four hours, can be reflected in your bowel habits.

Although physiological abnormalities or nerve damage can underlie constipation, the most frequent cause by far is poor diet; contributing factors are not enough water, and lack of exercise. No wonder that studies of constipation treatments have found that dietary changes make more difference than any other option! Frequently, especially in cases of constipation caused by irritable bowel syndrome, doctors may recommend that you add raw, unprocessed bran to your breakfast cereal. Just as you might when you first switch to a vegetarian diet, you may have gas and feel bloated until your digestive system adjusts. But your constipation will vanish if you turn to bran flakes, prune juice, and a high-fiber diet instead of reaching for laxatives. And even if you are trying to lose weight by avoiding fats, make sure that you put a few teaspoons of olive oil on your salad to prevent constipation.

Besides bran and fiber in general, dandelion or senna leaf tea, taken slowly in small doses, stimulates peristalsis and can work as an effective, safe laxative. You can also take a tablespoon of goldenseal, buckthorn bark, flax or linseed, or psyllium in a large glass of water. Bear in mind, however, that even herbal laxatives can be habit-forming. Only bulk-forming laxatives are entirely safe. Metamucil, whose main ingredient is psyllium in its refined form, is fine. Konsyl is even better because it contains unsweetened psyllium; Metamucil does include either sugar or aspartame, a sweetener marketed as NutraSweet. In season, in early summer, fresh rhubarb is a delicious and powerful antidote to constipation. Year round, you can turn to rhubarb extract in the form of pills or teas—unless you're prone to calcium kidney stones. Rhubarb's high oxalate content may give you more of them.

COLONICS: PRO AND CON

One of the few recommendations that conventional and alternative physicians both agree about nowadays is that fiber is crucial to your colon's proper functioning. Elsewhere, they part company—and nowhere more so than on the subject of colonics. Many doctors who practice alternative medicine believe that the normal Western diet—strong on junk food, fat, sugar, and meat—clogs your colon so that it never empties completely, even if you have frequent bowel movements. Fecal matter and mucus build up on its walls, and accumulate in tiny outpocketings called diverticula. As a result, colonics advocates say, your colon needs periodic cleansing with enemas and special diets to rid it of toxins that may fester and poison the rest of your body. The accumulated wastes also block your colon's ability to absorb nutrients, so that even if your diet is quite good, you can't reap its benefits. And the wastes can irritate the nerve endings in your colon, contributing to irritable bowel syndrome and other problems.

While most Americans rely on laxatives, some severely constipated people do turn to more time-consuming enemas to gently stretch the colon so that normal defecating reflexes can begin. Enemas have been used as a solution to constipation since ancient times, and periodically, up to the early twentieth century, they were very much in fashion. Colonics are more sophisticated and thorough enemas that gently cleanse your entire colon. Before you undergo colonics, you swallow an intestinal cleanser, usually made with psyllium or bentonite, a kind of volcanic ash, to help loosen stubborn fecal deposits. Then, during the painless half-hour procedure, your colon is repeatedly filled with distilled water or cold coffee made with it, through a tube inserted in your rectum. The water or coffee then empties out of your colon through this same tube. At the same time, you gently massage your abdomen. As the water or coffee washes out of your colon, any impacted mucus or fecal matter should come with it. Most colonics programs suggest weekly enemas for several months, and then once every three months as a preventive measure.

Colonics advocates speak of a feeling of lightness after a cleansing, along with renewed energy and relief of chronic constipation and related problems like frequent headaches. They also claim that a regular colon cleansing program can improve your general health and extend your life—often quite dramatically. One longtime advocate, V. E. Irons, is strong enough at 94 to go sailing on weekends! He says that he owes his longevity to following the example of Norman W. Walker, Ph.D., who established his own colon health clinic in 1910 and wrote a manual entitled *Colon Health: The Key to a Vibrant Life*. Another of Mr. Irons's mentors in colonics died recently, aged more than 100.

"I know it sounds hard to believe," Irons says, "but these deposits of fecal matter in your colon can get to be two to three inches thick and hard as a piece of black rubber that comes off a tire. Most colons are so twisted, clogged, and hardened with old feces that neither bran nor any other ordinary food roughage will unplug them. People never cease to be amazed at what they have been carrying around inside of them. There was one young lady who had been a vegetarian and light eater for over three years. She went on the program and was shocked to see all the material coming out of her. Afterwards she was almost five pounds lighter."

One of my colleagues, Dr. Kirk Zachary, a gastroenterologist who takes a preventive approach, has performed countless colonoscopies and certainly knows what a colon's interior usually looks like. He strongly disagrees with Irons's description, countering that "you never see accumulated material except in patients with diverticula"—out-pocketings of the colonic walls where fecal matter can be trapped. However, Irons might retort that as part of the preparation for a colonoscopy, you are given a purge, so that in reality, Dr. Zachary may be seeing the good results of colonics. Certainly, several patients who have undergone a colonoscopy have told me afterward, "Doctor, that was an awful procedure, but you know, I feel better—more alert, less sluggish."

Most conventional doctors take the position that this is nonsense. They say that colonics are totally unnecessary because they do not believe that your colon allows waste, sometimes pounds of it, as colonics enthusiasts maintain, to build up on its walls. Certainly, there are dangers when colonics are administered under unsanitary conditions or by uninformed technicians. In fact, there have been some appalling cases of colonics gone wrong. In 1982, a chiropractic clinic in Colorado had an outbreak of amebic infestation in its colonic irrigation reservoir that infected at least thirty-six clients—and killed seven. In a more recent case in New York City, a patient died on the colonic table. He had not been thoroughly screened before he underwent colonics; if he had been, the colonics therapist would have realized that his intestinal walls had been thinned by preexisting disease. As it happened, the enemas he was given had punctured them.

Scary as these stories are, they are a testament to shoddy approaches to colonics, not to the practice itself. In truth, more people have been injured or killed by colonoscopies, a standard method of examining your colon, than by colonics. Anyone who has a heart valve problem, or who has had heart valve surgery, is no candidate for colonics: you are much more vulnerable to bloodborne infections, and shouldn't undergo even a minor procedure like having your teeth cleaned without taking antibiotics. And you certainly should steer clear of colonics if you have severe hemorrhoids, colitis, a history of colon or rectal surgery or any kind of intestinal inflammation—even though V. E. Irons, among other advocates, would say otherwise. And too much enthusiasm for colonics can reflect a certain psychopathology: some people feel inordinately dirty, and the more they cleanse, the better off they think they are. This attitude is potentially quite harmful: if you use colonics too often, you may come to rely on them, just like laxatives.

I'm not opposed to colonics on an occasional basis, provided that you have had a complete physical examination recently, and your doctor has approved your plans for internal cleansing. Some doctors report amazing improvements in patients who have gone on a cleansing program. Make sure that you use distilled rather than chlorinated water, which kills your beneficial bacteria. As extra insurance, some colonics therapists advise lactobacillus "implants" in the water used during colonics.

Still, colonics amount to an extraordinary measure to correct chronic bowel problems. Because there is no government regulation of the colonics industry, there are no established standards of hygiene for colonics facilities. If you set out to find a reputable colonics therapist, *caveat emptor!* Adopting better diet habits and a regular exercise program will do you much more good in the long run.

Hemorrhoids

If laxatives are to blame for chronic constipation, then they are indirectly the chief cause of hemorrhoids, also known as piles, a painful side effect of constipation and straining to pass stool. They are a complaint as old as time: the ancient Egyptians, Babylonians, and Greeks had to put up with them. In the Middle Ages, people with hemorrhoids had their own patron saint, St. Fiacre, who—for reasons that may or may not be connected—also watches over gardeners. Napoleon suffered from piles on the battlefield. Imagine the agony of his retreat from Moscow on horseback—agony brought on by more than the sting of defeat.

Today, as many as half of all Americans have this painful condition by age 50. Hemorrhoids are extremely common during pregnancy, which can make defecating or even just sitting an excruciating experience. Hemorrhoids are veins around your rectum that tend to swell under pressure. These veins may be inside the rectum or under the skin around your anus. The main symptom of internal hemorrhoids is painless, bright-red bleeding when you defecate. Sometimes internal hemorrhoids protrude through your anus, and may or may not bleed.

External hemorrhoids are different from pruritus ani, or cracking, reddening and irritation of the skin around your anus. Pruritus ani is often due to a diet heavy in caffeine and spicy foods; I've noticed that a vegetarian regimen can bring relief. It also can be caused by stool that's highly alkaline—a sign of a deficiency of lactobacilli. Yogurt and lactobacillus supplements can help clear this condition.

Like pruritus ani, external hemorrhoids may bleed and they certainly itch. Until quite recently, surgery for severely painful hemorrhoids required anesthetic and a hospital stay, and was unbelievably uncomfortable. Then came two advances in hemorrhoid surgery: ligation and cryosurgery, simpler, less painful procedures that can be done in a doctor's office. Ligation involves using small rubber bands to tie off hemorrhoids, cutting off their supply of blood. Cryosurgery means freezing hemorrhoids, destroying the cells of their tissue. After either form of treatment, the hemorrhoids drop off within a week or two.

A new development is laser surgery. This is another brief, simple outpatient procedure that usually requires no anesthetic; infrared light is used to shrink hemorrhoids by causing them to clot and become reabsorbed into surrounding tissue. This method is popular in Europe. Over here, it certainly has not supplanted ligation or cryosurgery, but it is becoming more widely used.

If you don't want to have surgery—there is always a chance that hemorrhoids will reoccur after your operation—the best prescription for hemorrhoids and anal itching in general is bathing the area gently after defecating. Would that the bidet, that commodious feature of European hotel bathrooms, would catch on in America! We will have to get by with the clumsier and more time-consuming shower. Try to avoid vigorous wiping; use soft, moist toilet paper. If you are very uncomfortable, as you may be during or just after pregnancy, you can alternate warm sitz baths with cold ones or with ice packs.

There is another feature from other parts of the world that helps hemorrhoids: the very simple toilet that consists of two tile footprints with a hole between them. You stand on the footprints and squat to defecate. V. E. Irons believes that everyone—but especially if you suffer from hemorrhoids—should crouch or squat on the toilet, with both feet on the rim of the porcelain bowl, keeping your head forward. He says that in this position, "the colon straightens out, and your feces fall out so easily that pressure is relieved and your hemorrhoids begin to disappear." If Irons's idea catches on, there goes the comfortable habit of reading on the toilet! And it could be very disconcerting to watch someone's feet disappearing behind the locked door of a public toilet stall. Still, squatting is indeed more physiologically correct, and should ease any pain that hemorrhoids cause you when you void.

What about one of the most popular over-the-counter remedies of all, Preparation H? Or other suppositories and ointments for hemorrhoids? Unfortunately, they're usually useless. Some contain cortisone, which does ease itching and inflammation, but can have dangerous side effects if you use it constantly. Others contain benzocaine, an effective anesthetic that can cause allergic reactions. Studies have found that Preparation H helps heal open wounds, but hemorrhoids are not open wounds per se. There is no evidence that Preparation H can shrink swollen tissue, so it is not much help for hemorrhoids.

To ease itching and irritation, you can use petroleum jelly or zinc oxide cream or vitamin E suppositories. There are many herbs that can be made into soothing poultices or suppositories for hemorrhoids. One of the most effective is *Collinsonia canadensis,* or stoneroot, a herbal remedy which contains tannin, an astringent that can pucker the skin. You can also take it internally. Other useful herbs, some of which also contain tannin, are witch hazel, goldenseal, plantain, Solomon's seal, white oak bark, bayberry, yellow dock, yarrow, spearmint, comfrey, chickweed, wheatgrass, horse chestnut, and mullein.

But whether you choose surgery or another method of easing hemorrhoids, there is always a risk that they will recur unless you change your diet to soften your stool. Plenty of water and fiber is often all that's needed.

Irritable Bowel Syndrome

As many as 30 million Americans suffer the attacks of alternating diarrhea and constipation that characterize irritable bowel syndrome (IBS), also known as spastic colon or mucous colitis. This chronic bowel disorder, which usually begins in early adolescence, accounts for about half the visits people make to gastroenterologists. Irritable bowel syndrome, which mostly affects women, is an extremely frustrating condition: it can seem as elusive and hard to shake as a voodoo curse. You may endure years of abdominal bloating, nausea and pain, urgency that gets worse if you eat or are under stress, and a sensation of incomplete bowel movements. Classically, you seesaw back and forth between diarrhea and constipation, never feeling quite right.

You may spend a fortune on doctors and tests, only to be told that your colon shows no sign of any known disease. Meanwhile, irritable bowel syndrome may be ruining your life: three times a week, one of my patients had crippling pain that obliged her to go home, take off any clothes that put pressure on her lower abdomen, and lie down for several hours until the attack passed. If you suffer as much as she did, you may be very worried that sooner or later some doctor will discover that your condition has deteriorated, and now you *do* have an ulcer, colitis, or even cancer. The truth is that even severe cases of IBS rarely lead to true inflammatory disease.

Until very recently, however, that was cold comfort. Doctors used to suggest that, in the absence of signs of any true pathology, patients with chronic irritable bowel syndrome must have a psychosomatic illness, and ought to turn to psychotherapy or a program of stress reduction. These suggestions certainly weren't entirely off base: doctors were confused by the fact that many IBS patients do suffer from anxiety or depression—as well you might after years of pain that doesn't end and seems to have no cause!

Lately, there is new evidence that IBS starts, not in your head, but very definitely in your gut. Today, there is a new medical consensus that most patients with IBS are neither more depressed nor more anxious than their counterparts who are free of gastrointestinal symptoms.

Other people, who have different physiological Achilles' heels, might seek out back clinics or headache specialists. But IBS sufferers, because of abnormalities in the nervous system that serves their gastrointestinal tract, react to stress and upset with their guts. Your nerves and hormones direct electrical activity in your colon's muscles as they contract to propel their contents toward your rectum and to absorb water from feces. If you have IBS, the muscle in your lower colon contracts abnormally—something you experience as painful spasms, accompanied or followed by constipation or diarrhea.

There may be a genetic component to IBS: many of my patients have told me about other cases in their families. And some female sufferers turn out to have a kind of heart murmur called mitral valve prolapse, which is often associated with other autonomic nervous disorders like palpitations and "phantom" chest pain. Many IBS sufferers are particularly sensitive to bloating, and complain that they seem to have excessive amounts of gas. In reality, they simply are more sensitive to normal gas. When researchers inflated a small balloon in the intestines of IBS patients, they suffered spasms while others did not. The culprits most likely to trigger these abnormal contractions are diet and stress.

MEDICAL TREATMENT FOR IBS

IBS responds well to self-care, but you should consult your doctor as well, partly because this condition may mask parasitic infection or food intolerance. In any case, you especially need medical advice if you have certain symptoms, such as blood in the stool or persistent abdominal pain accompanied by a fever.

Thankfully, fiber has become a cornerstone of even the most orthodox treatment of IBS, because it helps relieve spasms and incomplete evacuation. Most physicians will suggest taking Metamucil or sprinkling raw bran on your breakfast cereal. Metamucil's main ingredient is psyllium seed, a soft soluble fiber that IBS patients seem to tolerate more easily. Coarse wheat bran may be too abrasive for sensitive colons, or may trigger allergies in some, negating fiber's benefits.

All too often, IBS treatment still relies heavily on powerful drugs, even though there is nothing available to cure it. Some drugs, like Lomotil or Imodium, mimic opium's bowel-quieting effects; others, like Donnatal, Bentyl, or Librax, are antispasmodics that slow intestinal contractions and relieve painful cramping. But most gastroenterologists regard these drugs as only sporadically effective, and they can have side effects like dryness of the mouth, impotence, and even glaucoma.

Sometimes IBS patients are also given antidepressants like Elavil or Sinequan, or antianxiety medications like Valium. Most of these drugs can cause side effects like dizziness, drowsiness or mental confusion, and—even worse—downright dependency. And they work by masking symptoms whose causes, with a little detective work, can be pinpointed and alleviated. IBS may have diverse causes, and each patient needs an individually tailored strategy of medical and self-care.

An important reason to see your doctor is to take a special test to make sure your symptoms are not really signs of the presence of harmful bacterial overgrowth or proliferating intestinal yeast. This is often the case if you have a history of antibiotics prescriptions, which could have upset the natural balance of your essential colonic bacteria, resulting in symptoms that seem to be IBS. You may need a prescription of an antifungal like nystatin to suppress fungal growth, as well as liberal doses of helpful bacteria in supplements or foods like yogurt, sauerkraut, or miso to restore your intestinal ecology.

Because conventional medicine frequently underestimates the prevalence of parasitic infections, they are often mistaken for IBS. Dr. Leo Galland, a New York internist, has used the mucus swab test to ferret out giardiasis. He has found that nearly a half of patients who seem to have IBS turn out to be infected with *Giardia*—and in three quarters of these cases, no doctor had previously considered that possibility. Dr. Galland estimates that in about a quarter of all IBS patients nationwide, the real culprit may be giardiasis.

Giardia is not the only parasite that can imitate IBS. Recently I treated a man who told me immediately that his problem was IBS, and had been for years. When I suggested the possibility of parasites, he shrugged. "You can test if you like, doctor, but I'm telling you, I have IBS." Sure enough, he turned out to be infected with *Blastocystis hominis,* a parasite once thought to be a harmless fellow traveler in the human intestine. Now it's recognized as a frequent culprit in chronic conditions ranging from irritable bowel syndrome to outright colitis. A quick course of antiparasitic medication eradicated this man's "IBS." For more on painless detection and treatment of parasites, see Week Six of the Hoffman Program.

If you have irritable bowel syndrome, you almost always have to make some changes in your diet. Your doctor can help you determine whether a particular one is necessary by testing you for lactose intolerance. The hereditary or acquired inability to break down lactose, or milk sugar, lactose intolerance can contribute to IBS. In 70 to 80 percent of nonwhites, lactose intolerance develops with age, and whites, particularly those of Mediterranean ancestry, are by no means exempt.

MAKING MORE CHANGES IN YOUR DIET

Many IBS patients tell me that they or their relatives have allergies or allergy-related conditions like asthma or arthritis. Researchers are beginning to recognize the connection between IBS and food intolerance. The foremost authorities on this subject, V. Alun Jones and his colleagues at Cambridge University in England, have written, "Although stress undoubtedly exacerbates IBS in some cases . . . food intolerance appears to be very important." This research team found that in two thirds of patients, specific foods provoke IBS symptoms. The most common culprits were wheat, corn, dairy products, coffee, tea, and citrus fruits.

If I suspect that any of these foods are troubling my patients, I suggest following an abbreviated form of my Pain-Stopper Diet for ten days (see pages 93–99). You eliminate all the food offenders implicated in IBS. After ten days, I find that about 40 percent of patients are distinctly better—and most of them don't even have to stay on a limited diet forever.

Rather, you can bring back each food you've eliminated, one by one. Eat each food for three successive days. To make sure that your test is accurate, eat the foods you are testing in whole forms. For example, if you are testing wheat, choose whole wheat matzoh, pita, or bulgur wheat, rather than whole wheat bread, which may consist of wheat plus corn syrup or barley malt, milk, eggs, yeast, and sometimes various preservatives.

Record the results of each three-day reintroduction, taking care to note in detail whether you have any symptoms. If you feel fine, you can eat that particular food with impunity; if you start to feel poorly again, then you know which one you cannot tolerate.

This mini-Pain-Stopper Diet will uncover any inability to tolerate lactose or gluten. Doctors used to think that gluten intolerance was quite rare, occurring only in patients who had unremitting diarrhea and who had lost their ability to absorb essential nutrients to the point where they had become dangerously emaciated. Today, new findings suggest that gluten intolerance, like many other forms of food intolerance, spans a clinical spectrum ranging from mild gas and abdominal bloating to severe, life-threatening digestive shutdown. If you have trouble digesting gluten, eliminating wheat and other grains that contain gluten from your diet may provide relief from IBS.

Fat intolerance can play a key part in triggering IBS because of fat's particular role in digestive physiology. In either vegetable or animal form, fat is the strongest stimulus of colonic contractions after a meal, prompting the urge to eliminate. That is the unhappy reason why many diners, out for a celebratory meal of buttery French haute cuisine, find themselves ending their special evening uncomfortably in the "Hommes" or "Dames." A digestive supplement containing lipase can help you digest fat properly.

ONE MAN'S THEORY

In the next chapter, when I discuss inflammatory bowel disease, I'll be talking more about De Lamar Gibbons, M.D., a general practitioner in Kellogg, Idaho, with a special interest in bowel problems. Based on his observations of his own patients, he believes that fructose, sorbitol, mannitol, and other sweeteners may cause just as many digestive problems as lactose does. Many people, he says, can't turn fructose into glucose and absorb it properly. Instead, fructose ferments in your large intestine, resulting in gas, cramps, loose stools, and the spasms of IBS.

I have urged several patients to adopt Dr. Gibbons's approach, suggesting that they eliminate fructose and other sugars for ten days, and thereafter limit themselves to one piece of fruit per day. Since sweets are a major form of having a good time, in diet terms, most people have trouble giving them up completely. And sugar and sweeteners are practically ubiquitous. Dr. Gibbons admits that he's advocating a pretty Spartan diet: there's sorbitol even in frankfurters, and corn syrup shows up in desserts, cereals, soda pop, and bottled salad dressings. He says most people go off his diet, get into digestive trouble, and in the process educate themselves about how far they can stray. One patient reported, "I cheat; I pay; I repent; I get back on your diet."

For occasional attacks of IBS, herbal remedies have proven remarkably effective. Peppermint, a smooth-muscle relaxant in the form of capsules of peppermint oil, is a mainstay of natural IBS care in Great Britain. In a 1984 study at the University Hospital of Wales, 83 percent of IBS sufferers felt that their symptoms had improved. Be sure that your capsules are enteric-coated, so that they will be released past your stomach, or you will be plagued with minty burps. Peppermint tea is carminative, meaning that it helps you expel excess gas. I also recommend Ileocecal Tonic, which contains several herbs—quassia, bistort, ginger, angelica, bayberry—that stop spasms by relaxing your ileocecal valve, on the right-hand side of your lower abdomen, connecting your small and large intestines. Some patients tell me that a few drops of this tonic in peppermint or chamomile tea work faster than any drug they've ever tried.

SOOTHING STRESS

Since stress can trigger uncomfortable spasms, psychotherapy and relaxation techniques like exercise, massage, biofeedback, meditation, and even hypnotherapy can help alleviate IBS. A recent study shows that hypnosis can relieve IBS symptoms in over 50 percent of sufferers. Acupuncture has also been successful in relieving IBS pain. (See Week Seven of the Hoffman Program for more about relaxation techniques, and see the description of the principles of acupuncture in this sidebar.) Some doctors have reported striking improvements in IBS patients who have embarked on meditation programs. All these practices prompt the release of endorphins, your body's own internal tranquilizers and pain relievers.

HOW ACUPUNCTURE WORKS

Acupuncture is a form of therapy invented in China some 4,000 years ago. Continuously practiced in China and Japan, it spread in the early twentieth century to Europe, where it is quite widespread, and to the United States. Americans did not become widely acquainted with acupuncture until 1972, during President Richard Nixon's visit to China, when *New York Times* columnist
(continued on page 206)

(continued from page 205)

James Reston described his acupuncture treatment after an attack of appendicitis.

In the early 1970s, numerous American and European doctors and medical students flocked to China to study acupuncture and traditional Chinese medicine. At first, in the United States, there was a good deal of opposition from the conventional medical establishment. When Nevada decided to license acupuncturists, the *Journal of the American Medical Association* condemned acupuncture as a "two-armed bandit."

Small wonder: while Western medicine takes an analytical approach, diagnosing and treating the body as a mechanism, Chinese medicine regards it as an energy field. Until quite recently, most Western physicians dismissed acupuncture as a philosophical approach to the body, rather than a scientific one. According to acupuncture theory, a patient is a microcosm of the universe, with two major forces, yin and yang, affecting his or her balance of energy, or *chi*. When chi is out of balance, the patient is ill. A Chinese physician has to find the deficiencies or blockages that create imbalance. He does so by palpitating and interpreting twelve different pulses and by examining the patient's tongue, which reflects the body's internal condition. You can test this form of diagnosis yourself: If you aren't feeling well, your tongue is likely to be coated, yellowish, creamy or even spotted instead of a smooth rosy pink.

Because every patient is different, acupuncture is a highly individualized treatment. For instance, while a Western doctor would consider a peptic ulcer a single diagnostic category, Chinese medicine recognizes six subtypes in every category of digestive disorder, according to the patient's balance of energy toward "heat" or "cold." Depending on the diagnosis, the doctor inserts one or more thin, fine needles—this is rarely any more painful than a mosquito bite—into one or more of 400 acupuncture points. All these points are both diagnostic and therapeutic. They are located on your head, trunk, and limbs on twelve paired and two unpaired major meridians, or hypothetical lines of force, that supposedly traverse your body from head to toe. The insertion of needles—sometimes with painless electrical stimulus as well—is thought to move energy and adjust imbalance.

Recently, the Western view of acupuncture has become more favorable, mainly because the procedure often works—with al-

(continued from opposite page)

most no pain and no side effects. Moreover, both Chinese and Western researchers have devoted themselves successfully to establishing scientific explanations for acupuncture's effectiveness. They have established that acupuncture stimulates your immune system and blocks pain by releasing endorphins, your body's natural tranquilizers and anesthetics. Acupuncture also triggers the release of cortisone from your adrenal gland, helping to promote healing. One prominent acupuncture researcher, Dr. Bruce Pomeranz, speculates that since the hole made by an acupuncture needle stays open for twenty-four hours, this tiny wound also encourages healing.

Today, nearly 6,000 doctors and other medical professionals practice acupuncture in this country. Probably the most dramatic and well-publicized application of acupuncture has been to relieve addicts' pain as they withdraw from alcohol and drugs, including crack. But practitioners also report success using acupuncture to treat a variety of chronically painful digestive disorders, including hemorrhoids, nausea, diarrhea, morning sickness, irritable bowel syndrome, and ulcerative colitis. Dr. Gabriel Stux, who heads the German Acupuncture Society and runs an acupuncture clinic in Dusseldorf, has used acupuncture to relax gastrointestinal motility and anesthetize patients during colonoscopies and endoscopies. And Dr. William Chey, a gastroenterologist at Genesee Hospital in Rochester, New York, has noticed that acupuncture has encouraged esophageal motility in a patient with a ''nutcracker esophagus'' that caused her great difficulty in swallowing.

You can apply acupuncture yourself: one of the most effective and widely used acupuncture points, *hegu,* is at the base of your thumb. Not coincidentally, your thumb, of all your digits and limbs, has the largest collection of nerves and connections to your brain. *Hegu* is a key point for diagnosing problems in its corresponding organ, the colon. If you don't feel well, or have a headache—many headaches are due to constipation or other gastrointestinal problems—try gripping the base of your thumb with your other thumb and forefingers. If something has gone wrong in your large intestine, this pressure will produce dull pain at this acupuncture point. And if you decide to go to an acupuncturist, he or she will treat you by inserting needles in *hegu.*

Many experienced sailors are familiar with another acupuncture point, located about one hand's span above your wrist, be-

(continued on page 208)

(continued from page 207)

tween the two tendons on the inner surface of your forearm. By pressing hard on this point, you can overcome seasickness. In fact, a recent catalog of exclusive and expensive goods offered a special yachting bracelet that, when fastened, applied continuous pressure on this acupuncture point.

A word of caution about one form of exercise: as I've already mentioned, running can bring on reflux and heartburn. Some IBS sufferers also find that it can trigger spasms, especially if you run just after a meal. And running does not strengthen your abdominal muscles, the very muscles that need toning if you have IBS. Most helpful are exercises such as crunches and sit-ups, or yoga exercises to improve peristalsis.

Just as it's important to keep track of *what* you eat when you have IBS, it's crucial to be aware of *how* you eat. I've already talked about the fact that eating and chewing slowly are key to good digestion. Since eating can trigger abnormal contractions in your colon, eating slowly is doubly important for anyone with irritable bowel syndrome. If you look around a table and consistently find that you're the first to finish your meal, either you're not contributing enough to the conversation —or you're eating too fast.

New Approaches
to Serious
Digestive Problems

"The serpent is in man; it is the intestines. It tempts, betrays, and punishes."

—Victor Hugo

Whenever you feel acute abdominal pain, you may wonder, at least in passing, whether anything is badly wrong with you. Perhaps you've just eaten something that has disagreed with you—but then again, perhaps you have appendicitis, or your minor, chronic problem has worsened into something that's more than annoying. If you do find that you need treatment for a severe gastrointestinal difficulty, here are some new approaches and treatments that will help you get the best possible care.

Appendicitis

Appendicitis probably is completely preventable: a century ago, before refined foods were widespread, it was a rarity in Western countries, and it is still very unusual among peoples who eat a high-fiber diet. If you do have appendicitis, and it is not treated promptly and properly, it can be life-threatening. Unfortunately, appendicitis is often mistaken for other problems, and vice versa. You may pass off the pain of appendicitis as gas. Several diseases, including inflammation of the gallbladder, ulcers, intestinal obstructions, diverticulitis, uterine problems, kidney infections, and even heart disease, pneumonia or shingles, can have symptoms that closely resemble appendicitis. I've mentioned the case of a young man who was operated on for appendicitis, but who turned out to have a severe parasitic infection, thanks to a serving of homemade sushi.

Appendicitis means that your appendix, a small, dead-end sac attached to your large intestine at the point where it joins your small intestine, has become inflamed. This can happen much more frequently in teenagers and young adults than in people over 50, and somewhat more often in men than in women. As your meal is broken down in your stomach and partially absorbed in your small intestine, some of it may work its way into your appendix en route to your colon. Usually peristalsis keeps intestinal contents moving on their way. But if the appendix's lining is swollen or if its opening is blocked by undigested particles like seeds, then more swelling and infection may set in. If your appendix ruptures under the extra pressure, and bacteria spill into your peritoneal cavity, you may come down with peritonitis, a very serious, even fatal condition.

Appendicitis usually starts with pain around your navel that may feel just like gas. But appendicitis pain persists, and is usually accompanied by a low fever as well as nausea and vomiting—because your infection is preventing normal digestion. Your lower right abdomen may feel painfully tender, and a cough, sneeze, or any jarring movement may make this tenderness worse. If you suspect you have appendicitis, you should not eat, and above all, you should not take laxatives. Because laxatives increase peristalsis and muscle activity in your intestines, they may make rupture more likely by blocking the protective mechanisms that can wall off your infection.

ANOTHER VIEW OF APPENDECTOMIES

Because of this risk of rupture, most doctors who suspect you have appendicitis want to operate and remove your appendix. This is quite understandable and advisable, but many doctors are also prone to use other operations as an excuse to take out your perfectly healthy appendix, under the impression that they're doing you a favor. The conventional medical view is that your appendix serves no useful purpose in digestion, so it's no surprise that appendectomies are the fifth most common surgical procedure in this country, and that about a quarter of the population has had a normal appendix removed. Here's how appendectomies often happen: Suppose you're obliged to have a hysterectomy or a gallbladder operation. Your surgeon may tell you, "By the way, we nipped out that appendix—just to save you trouble later." This "bonus" not only is unnecessary; it may be quite dangerous. Your appendix is made of lymphatic tissue, so it is part of your digestive system's immune system. Some researchers report a higher rate of lymphatic cancer in people who have had appendectomies. So unless your appendix is already inflamed, you may be better off if you keep it.

Most surgeons feel that resorting to antibiotics to treat appendicitis is risky because important symptoms may be obscured; early removal of the appendix, they maintain, is much safer. But Dr. George Crile, former chief of surgery at the prestigious Cleveland Clinic, differs radically in his view of appendectomy. Dr. Crile has successfully treated cases of appendicitis, even some patients whose appendix had already ruptured, with antibiotics only. Afterward, he became "convinced that appendectomy was not a necessary or even an effective treatment for appendicitis" if antibiotics were available. Nevertheless, the broad consensus of modern surgical opinion is still in favor of appendectomies.

Diarrhea

Diarrhea is the opposite of constipation: while constipation means that your bowel movements are too infrequent and you pass them with difficulty, diarrhea means that they are very frequent and too loose. Diarrhea can be chronic: when it lasts for weeks or even months, sometimes accompanied by a fever, it is a sign of serious illness— perhaps colitis or some form of intestinal cancer. Or it means that parasites, such as amoebas or *Giardia*, have taken up residence in your bowel. In either case, you need prompt medical attention.

Acute diarrhea is different: almost everyone has a bout once in a while—three or four days of diarrhea, perhaps accompanied by nausea and vomiting. This kind of attack is just about the most common reason people call in sick to work. People rarely bother to go to the doctor with acute diarrhea, tending to blame it on something they ate. They say, "It must have been that apple pie—it ran right through me." This *can* be true: diarrhea is a frequent symptom of food allergy or intolerance. A meal can also trigger your gastrocolic reflex. Almost as soon as you have eaten, this reflex flashes a signal to your large intestine, and you are forced to rush to the nearest toilet. But unless you cannot tolerate lactose, or have irritable bowel syndrome, this reflex is usually lost after infancy.

Basically, when you have acute diarrhea, you have an attack of food poisoning or an infection caused by a virus or bacteria. In most people, this short siege of bowel infection is not serious and passes quickly. But in infants, who, like the elderly and people with major illnesses, are particularly vulnerable to bowel infections, diarrhea can be fatal. In the United States, the Centers for Disease Control have found, diarrhea kills hundreds of infants every year, mostly among the poor, especially in the South. And in the Third World, diarrhea is the major killer of children: about 4.5 million die from it annually.

Especially in its chronic form, diarrhea can be dangerous because you lose water and salt, which can lead to dehydration. Your normal stool is 60 percent water. When you have diarrhea, your stool weighs more, reflecting more water being excreted rather than reabsorbed. If you have a viral or bacterial infection, your bowel is irritated and pours out water. The abnormally rapid transit that accompanies diarrhea means that your gut has no time to absorb your food properly, so you're also deprived of nutrients. Anyone who has chronic, wasting diarrhea risks malnutrition.

BE A DIGESTIVE SLEUTH: CHECK OUT THE CAUSES
OF YOUR DIARRHEA

Diarrhea is not a disease in itself, but a symptom of many different problems, some serious, some minor. To determine what is causing yours, here are some questions to consider:

• *How long has your bout been going on?* If you've been suffering less than a week, chances are you have acute diarrhea that will pass soon. Recurring but sporadic diarrhea can be a symptom of irritable bowel syndrome, especially if your diarrhea occurs when you're under stress or if it alternates with constipation. If diarrhea lasts ten days or longer, you should see a doctor in case something is seriously wrong.

• *What are your stools like?* Are you sure you have diarrhea? Some people assume that very loose, very frequent stools spell diarrhea, but diarrhea is usually quite different. If your stools are not only frequent but definitely watery and voluminous, you have diarrhea.

• *Is your diarrhea bloody?* If you have a short bout of acute diarrhea with some blood, your problem may be hemorrhoids. But if you have chronic diarrhea that's bloody, you may have colitis or a parasitic infection—or even cancer. In any case, see a doctor.

• *Do you have a fever?* If your diarrhea is accompanied by a temperature, even only a slight one, you may have the flu, or you may have appendicitis. Call your doctor if it persists.

• *Have you gone camping or hiking, or traveled abroad recently?* You may have picked up an infection, especially if you drank fresh water from a lake or stream. If your diarrhea won't go away, you may have parasites and should be tested. If your diarrhea lasts only a few days, you probably have traveler's diarrhea, a sign that you've come into contact with unfamiliar bacteria. Your symptoms will clear up once you return home, or if you remain abroad until your gut adjusts. For more about parasitic infections and traveler's diarrhea, see Week Six of the Hoffman Program and also the next chapter.

• *Are you expecting your period?* If you have irritable bowel syndrome or endometriosis—some women have both—you may have painful periods heralded or accompanied by diarrhea. It generally lasts only as long as your period.

• *Do you have diarrhea after you eat certain foods?* Perhaps you've picked out something spoiled. Diarrhea also is a common sign of food allergy or intolerance. If milk, ice cream, and other dairy products seem to bring on diarrhea, you may have lactose intolerance. If the culprit is usually whole wheat bread, you may not be able to tolerate gluten. And if the price of eating fine French cuisine is usually "the runs," you probably cannot tolerate fat.

• *Do those you live or work with have diarrhea, too?* You all may have food poisoning from eating the same contaminated food. Parasites or bacteria like *Salmonella*, *E. coli*, and *Campylobacter* may lurk in eggs, poultry, dairy products like cheese or mayonnaise, fish and shellfish. For more on food poisoning, see the next chapter.

• *Do you have a serious illness?* AIDS, AIDS-related complex (ARC), diabetes, cystic fibrosis, or a carcinoid tumor can cause diarrhea. But unless you are at risk for any of these diseases, a bout of diarrhea shouldn't prompt you to jump to the worst possible conclusion.

• **Does your infant or child have frequent diarrhea?** Because breast milk confers some protection against intestinal infections, infants who are exclusively breast-fed have diarrhea much less frequently than babies who are fed formula. But if you are breast-feeding and have been drinking cow's milk, and your baby is allergic to cow's milk, he or she will have diarrhea. Or the problem could be apple juice: recent studies have found that children have a limited ability to absorb fructose, and apple juice's fructose content is very high. Pear juice can also cause diarrhea because it is high in sorbitol. And if your baby is colicky and has diarrhea as well, he or she may be suffering from irritable bowel syndrome—now recognized as a remarkably frequent disorder in children, too. Do your children spend time in day care? *Giardia*, bacterial, and viral infections—all major causes of diarrhea—can spread rapidly through a center. For more about children's intestinal problems, see the next chapter.

• **What vitamins or supplements are you taking?** Yes, you *can* have too much of good things: large amounts of vitamin C, fish oil supplements, calcium citrate, or any magnesium supplements can give you diarrhea. And too much fiber can have the same unhappy result.

• **Are you taking any drugs?** Some antibiotics and antacids, as well as any laxative, notably milk of magnesia, can give you diarrhea. So can some drugs that dissolve gallstones, excessive amounts of thyroid medication, and drugs used as part of chemotherapy for cancer.

• **Have you had gastrointestinal surgery recently?** If your surgery has caused malabsorption or "dumping syndrome," you will have chronic diarrhea.

• **Are you on a diet?** If you are trying to lose weight by eating large amounts of dietetic foods, you may be downing quite a bit of sorbitol. Since this form of sugar can't be absorbed, it may be giving you diarrhea.

• **Do you have more than two drinks daily?** Too much wine, beer, or hard liquor can cause diarrhea. This is a major reason why alcohol abusers usually suffer from malnutrition.

TREATING DIARRHEA

Most cases of acute diarrhea clear up on their own. In fact, studies have shown that overtreating diarrhea with antibiotics and anti-diarrheal medications has actually prolonged certain kinds of infectious diarrhea. For infectious diarrhea, the most popular over-the-counter medications include bismuth, the main ingredient in Pepto-Bismol, which can turn your stool black but does diminish loss of water from your intestines, and may give you some protection from microorganisms that are causing your diarrhea. Both Imodium A-D, whose main ingredient is loperamide, and Lomotil can halt diarrhea by slowing down peristalsis in your intestine, allowing more time for waste to absorb water.

Clay, like the mixture of kaolin and pectin in Kaopectate, makes your stool bulkier, and may absorb and trap microorganisms and toxins. Bentonite, a volcanic ash like kaolin, can be mixed with distilled water into another clay that alleviates diarrhea. Paradoxically, bentonite is also an effective laxative, and in the Soviet Union, it has been used to treat peptic ulcers. Another natural remedy is blackberry root or blackberry cordial, whose astringency tends to close your loose bowels. Chinese medicine prescribes an aromatic combination of cinnamon and peony. For acute diarrhea, I've borrowed from pediatricians a dietary regime with the acronym BRAT: it consists of bananas, (white) rice, applesauce, and (herbal) tea, preferably chamomile. Acidophilus supplements also help relieve severe diarrhea.

If you are obliged to take a drug that is giving you diarrhea temporarily, avoid most dairy products, which can aggravate diarrhea, and choose foods containing pectin, such as apples or applesauce, and potassium, such as bananas. Avoid gas-producing food, raw salads, fruit and vegetable juices, carbonated beverages, and caffeine. Try eating your food lukewarm; hot food increases transit time, and makes your stool looser. On the other hand, if you are already taking a drug, and come down with diarrhea, you should be aware that diarrhea can interfere with proper absorption of most drugs, including birth control pills.

Surprisingly, researchers have found that some dairy products, most of which make diarrhea worse, can actually help clear it up. One of them is whey, the liquid left after milk has been made into cheese. Whey is a mainstay of Ayurvedic medicine, the traditional medicine of India. In the fourth century B.C., Hippocrates frequently prescribed whey, especially for acute septic conditions. Whey remained a popular medication throughout the Middle Ages. Today it is mostly used as a stabilizer and emulsifier in ice cream, beer, and various processed foods, but it is also an ingredient in Amish whey cheese, yogurt, and sour cream.

Recently, a Canadian study found that besides providing you with calcium and other nutrients, whey seems to boost immunity and help you fight infections, including the ones that cause diarrhea. The whey in breast milk helps a suckling infant resist intestinal infections, and promotes the growth of at least one variety of beneficial bacteria. Metagenics, a small California company, is trying to patent and market Probioplex, made of whey protein concentrate, to forestall intestinal infections that may give you diarrhea.

Another milk product that helps chronic diarrhea is a special form of bovine or human colostrum, the substance that appears before milk when a nursing infant begins to suck. Colostrum is rich in antibodies and other substances that fight intestinal infections. Hyperimmune bovine colostrum—that is, colostrum from an animal intentionally infected with a small dose of an intestinal parasite, virus, or bacteria—has been used successfully in Australia to treat chronic diarrhea. In New York City, there has been some limited experimentation using hyperimmune colostrum to treat AIDS patients. They often die of malnutrition because their lowered intestinal resistance to harmful organisms allows chronic, wasting diarrhea to develop.

There are also several new—but strictly experimental—treatments for chronic diarrhea that involve implanting substances through your rectum into your colon. One is ozone, the main gas in smog and in the layer above the earth's atmosphere that protects us from the sun's harmful ultraviolet rays. Until recently, only holistic practitioners in Europe ever used ozone as part of medical treatment. But in 1988, a study at the Veterans Administration Medical Center in San Francisco found that when ozone was administered rectally to AIDS patients so that it could be absorbed quickly into the blood, it stopped the AIDS virus from multiplying. After three or four administrations, it also relieved diarrhea. At present, as far as conventional medicine is concerned, the jury is still out on this procedure, as researchers continue to investigate its purported benefits.

At the University of Nebraska, Dr. Khem Shahani, who has carried out extensive research with lactobacilli, has found that lactobacillus supplements or implants in your colon can help clear up infectious diarrhea. He reasons that before this type of diarrhea can start, some pathogenic bacteria colonize your gut, spreading in number so that your beneficial bacteria, such as lactobacilli, are crowded out. Taking extra lactobacilli restores your gut's ecology. Besides, these bacteria

---

When You Need More Help

also can help inhibit the growth of invading bacteria, so that your diarrhea ceases.

Danish researchers have used another method of restoring colonic balance. Since your feces contain the right mix of friendly bacteria in your colon, they suspected that patients with chronic diarrhea caused by excessive use of antibiotics might improve if their colons were implanted with an analogous mixture of bacteria from a healthy person's feces. So in one case, a patient received a small, carefully introduced inoculation of bacteria from feces donated by a healthy relative. Five others were given rectal infusions that mimicked the mix of bacteria in their own feces. Sure enough, the patients' colonic balance of bacteria was restored, and the six patients recovered. This approach sounds promising, but because of the danger of introducing harmful organisms into a patient's colon, it is certainly not a measure to be undertaken lightly.

Ulcers

Up to 12 percent of Americans have ulcers at some point in life. Peptic ulcers are sores found in the lining of your stomach or of your duodenum, the upper portion of your small intestine. Duodenal ulcers are the more common, accounting for three quarters of all cases. Ulceration occurs when the stomach's or duodenum's mucosal lining cannot withstand the corrosive action of gastric juice, which your stomach's lining secretes to break down your meals. Gastric juice, which consists of hydrochloric acid and an enzyme, pepsin, which breaks down protein, can digest any living tissue, including your stomach and duodenum. Normally, both your stomach and duodenum are bathed constantly in gastric acid. But protective mechanisms, including the work of prostaglandins, which govern secretion of mucus from your stomach lining, and your food and saliva's ability to dilute acid, prevent your stomach from digesting itself.

In the past few years, medical thinking about peptic ulcers has changed dramatically: doctors used to think that having ulcers meant that you produced too much gastric acid. Some people with duodenal ulcers do secrete abnormal amounts of acid, but as many as half do not. And in most cases of gastric or stomach ulcers, acid is normal or even reduced. Now researchers recognize that the causes are more complex, and may include a failure of your stomach's cytoprotection.

Other contributing factors may be smoking, alcohol, family predisposition, emotional stress, and even bacterial infection or the use of common pain-killing medications like aspirin.

Peptic ulcers are chronic; they may recur at any time. Ulcers are rarely a prelude to cancer, but some ulcers, especially gastric ulcers, are an erosion of the stomach due to cancer. Even if ulcers are not cancerous, they can be very dangerous. An untreated ulcer can cause intestinal obstruction or rapid bleeding into your intestinal tract, which can be fatal. And like a ruptured appendix, an ulcer that erodes all the way through the wall of your stomach or duodenum can cause peritonitis. If you have an ulcer and any of these complications set in, you may need surgery. Thankfully, because of new drugs, ulcer surgery has become relatively rare. Certainly there are some steps you can take to avoid such a dire solution to ulcers.

FUELING AN ULCER'S FIRE

The first sign of an ulcer may be a good deal of belching and bloating, so that you may think you have a bad case of gas pains. But the pain becomes sharp and constant, and sometimes feels like a "stitch" somewhere between your navel and the base of your breastbone. It may be particularly gnawing between meals, or when your stomach is empty; you feel some relief after you eat something—but perplexingly, the reverse can also be true. Even after an ulcer heals, you may feel pain in that portion of your gut if you eat or drink anything that irritates your stomach lining. One woman in her early thirties who had had a duodenal ulcer felt this "weak link" act up when she had morning sickness during pregnancy and whenever she drank carbonated beverages, even decaffeinated ones, or alcohol on an empty stomach.

As far as we know, moderate consumption of alcohol and caffeine doesn't cause ulcers. But alcohol and caffeine do stimulate acid secretion in your stomach, as does decaffeinated coffee. Caffeine also blocks production of prostaglandins, weakening your stomach's cytoprotection. So any of these ingredients of popular beverages can exacerbate an ulcer you already have. Surprisingly, so can milk, which used to be a mainstay of ulcer patients' diets. Initially, milk does neutralize stomach acid—but then, acting on the rebound, it prompts the production of even more. Stress may not cause ulcers as frequently as most doctors once thought, but it can increase pain or flare-ups. One Australian study found that duodenal ulcers frequently recur when patients go through marital separation or divorce. Genes and gender also may contribute to ulcers: You're three times as likely to get an ulcer if any of your relatives have them. Men get twice as many duodenal ulcers, while the rate of gastric ulcers is about the same in both sexes.

Smoking—even chewing nicotine gum—certainly does cause ulcers. In fact, smoking not only doubles your risk of coming down with an ulcer, but slows its healing and contributes to recurrence. If you quit smoking and take no medication at all, your ulcer will heal more quickly than if you down drugs conscientiously but continue to smoke. Another sure cause of ulcers is regular use of aspirin and other nonsteroidal antiinflammatory medications like Motrin or Advil. Arthritis patients are particularly apt to take these drugs habitually over a long period of time. But aspirin and similar medications inhibit your stomach's production of prostaglandins, which are the key substances for cytoprotection. Prostaglandins govern mucus secretion and other mechanisms that protect your stomach's mucosal lining from injury by gastric juice, as well as other chemicals. If you stop taking the offending medications, your ulcers usually clear up. A new ulcer drug, Cytotec, offers your stomach cytoprotection even if you're obliged to take aspirin or other pain medications. But Cytotec has some side effects, ranging from the annoying (diarrhea) to the downright dangerous (miscarriages).

Many medications prescribed for "acid conditions" can actually add to your misery. Many doctors and patients, assuming that too much stomach acid equals ulcers, rely on antacids. This can make as much sense as putting out a fire while simultaneously relighting it. One popular antacid, Alka-Seltzer, contains aspirin, so large doses can actually cause ulcers. Another common antacid ingredient, calcium carbonate, found in Tums, can constipate you. And three or four hours after you take it, calcium carbonate stimulates increased gastric secretion.

Specific ulcer drugs, like best-selling Zantac and Tagamet, seem to suppress symptoms without clearing up the problem. Most patients who take them relapse within two years. These drugs work by blocking production of stomach acid. That may relieve your pain dramatically, but can be harmful in the long run. A certain level of acid secretion is necessary to digest proteins properly and to absorb vitamins and minerals. So if you're taking an ulcer drug, you may be setting the stage for malabsorption. Stomach acid also protects you by killing fungi, bacteria, and viruses that you cannot help ingesting along with your food. Without gastric acid's protection, you may be much more susceptible to food poisoning, parasites, and other gastrointestinal afflictions—including ulcers.

CAN YOU CATCH AN ULCER?

According to recent medical research, one reason ulcers tend to run in families is that they could be the result of infection with a particular bacterium, *Campylobacter pylori,* which certainly does cause gastritis. Investigators have noticed that most ulcers occur in the presence of gastric secretion that most people can tolerate easily. And many ulcers heal without any decrease in gastric acid output—a sure sign that gastric secretions are not the primary cause of ulcers, and that some other factor is at work.

Dr. Barry J. Marshall, an Australian researcher, is convinced that *C. pylori* is at the bottom of most cases of duodenal ulcers, as well as 70 percent of gastric ulcers and about half of all cases of dyspepsia without ulcers. Many patients infected with *C. pylori* whom Dr. Marshall has seen started with gastritis that developed into dyspepsia or peptic ulcers. In 1984, Dr. Marshall tested his own hypothesis by downing a potion of *C. pylori.* Sure enough, he got gastritis, a common precursor of ulcers. Marshall believes that the bacterium protects itself from hydrochloric acid, and also frequently eludes detection by burrowing beneath your stomach's protective mucosa.

Marshall also has been testing his theory by screening ulcer patients' families for infection with *C. pylori.* His team has found that the bacterium often spreads to ulcer patients' spouses and family members. This transmission, not heredity, may explain why ulcers run in families. Detecting *C. pylori* involves analyzing a sample of the patient's stomach lining, which means that he or she has to undergo an endoscopy. I have used a blood test, which is somewhat less reliable, but also less invasive and less expensive.

At this point, there is no perfect antidote to *C. pylori* infection. Bismuth, a metallic element that is a main ingredient in Pepto-Bismol, does seem to kill off the bug. In Australia, one study reported that 92 percent of duodenal ulcer patients healed after being treated with an antibiotic and a drug containing bismuth. After a year, only 21 percent had relapsed. This is how Dr. Marshall cleared up his self-induced gastritis. Antibiotics can exacerbate gastrointestinal symptoms—so much so that the treatment may be worse than the disease. Marshall would like to find a better solution—perhaps a vaccine.

THE HOFFMAN ULCER DIET

For years, ulcer patients had to survive on a bland diet of boiled fish, rice, milk, and cream. Now we know that while milk coats your stomach and may relieve your ulcer pain temporarily, it may retard your ulcer's healing. The calcium in milk can make you feel worse in the long run by stimulating the production of gastric acid. So can fried foods, citrus fruits, alcohol, caffeine in beverages or in chocolate, decaffeinated coffee, and smoking. Tea seems to particularly stimulate production of gastric juice. In case your ulcer is due to a food intolerance or allergy, try ferreting offenders out with an elimination diet, or ask a doctor who is knowledgeable about nutrition for the appropriate tests. And go through your medicine cabinet and throw out all aspirin and other nonsteroidal analgesics. Here are some other measures to consider:

• *Take Things Slower:* If you eat fast, bolting down your meals on the run, you're probably tense and thus more prone to indigestion. Try slowing down at the table—and in life in general: your response to stress can make a big difference in how quickly ulcers heal. One particular stress management technique, hypnotherapy, has helped 50 percent of patients suffering from duodenal ulcers.

• *Chili Medicine:* The old bland regimen that ulcer patients had to follow precluded spices like chili pepper, black pepper, mustard, cloves, and paprika. But recent studies in Texas and India indicate that this restriction may not always be necessary, and could be counterproductive. The Texas study found that eating jalapeño peppers did not harm gastric mucosa—even when ground peppers were placed directly in patients' stomachs! In the Indian study, fifty duodenal ulcer patients were fed a diet that included a gram of red chili powder (cayenne pepper) added to each meal. The researchers were trying to approximate the average Indian's daily intake of spices. Patients who ate chili powder healed just as quickly as patients who got no spice. Although hot peppers are very popular throughout India, ulcers are no more common than in other countries. If ulcers are indeed the result of a bacterial infection, then spices may confer some protection because they stimulate production of gastric juice, which fights bacteria. So unless you find spices irritate your gut, there's no need to cut them out while your ulcer heals.

• *Fiber Heals:* A high-fiber diet (high in unrefined grains, raw nonacidic fruit and vegetables) seems to heal ulcerous and preulcerous conditions much better than the old-fashioned bland diet. You can keep one part of the old diet, rice—although brown rice is better because it contains more fiber. Ulcer patients who go on a high-fiber diet find that their ulcers recur half as frequently. Barley, oats, and kudzu, a starch made from a root popular in Japanese and macrobiotic cooking, are especially helpful because they are mucilaginous: they coat and soothe your stomach lining. A high-fiber diet also will speed transit time, reducing gastritis. Avoid abrasive roughage like nuts, popcorn, and seeds.

• *Cut Down on Steak:* Animal proteins are high in arachidonic acid, a fatty acid used in your body's production of inflammatory prostaglandins. (Helpful prostaglandins derived from fish oil have an opposite, antiinflammatory effect.) If you can, try a vegetarian diet, at least temporarily: it will help reduce inflammation, as it does in other conditions like rheumatoid arthritis.

• *Choose Cabbage Juice:* If you down about a quart of cabbage juice daily, studies have found, your ulcer will heal more rapidly. Cabbage juice is high in substances that protect your gut's mucous-membrane lining, including L-glutamine, an amino acid, and gefarnate, which stimulates the secretion of mucus from your stomach's lining. You can make your own cabbage juice in a juicer or grinder. But since cabbage's ulcer-fighting powers vary greatly, depending on growing conditions, choose only fresh green cabbages; the best ones are spring and summer cabbages. Celery juice also contains factors that help heal ulcers.

• *Drink Plenty of Water:* I've described water's beneficial effect on digestion in general. Plenty of water—especially cold water, which feels soothing—seems to be particularly helpful if you have ulcers. An Iranian doctor who was detained in jail for two and a half years treated over 3,000 prisoners who had ulcer symptoms, from the stress of incarceration and bad treatment at the hands of their jailors. The doctor found that, in most cases, a glass of water relieved ulcer pains within three to eight minutes. Patients with particularly severe pain sometimes required two glasses. For the duration of the experiment, patients drank a glass of water a half-hour before and two and a half hours after each meal to prevent recurrences. Water was all these patients got; antacids or other ulcer medications were not available, and didn't seem necessary.

• *Prefer Plantains:* Unripe plantain bananas, a folk remedy for ulcers that can be taken in the form of dried extract, counteract the ulcerous effects of aspirin, and help heal ulcers you already have. Plantains contain a substance which stimulates healing of gastric mucosa.

• *Stock Up on Vitamins:* If you have an ulcer, you may also have signs of vitamin or mineral deficiency: perhaps your night vision has deteriorated, or you have sudden cramps in your legs in the middle of the night. Vitamins A, B_6, and E and folic acid also help maintain and repair your gut's mucosal barrier. Zinc supplements have healed ulcers, probably because zinc is necessary for vitamin A stored in your liver to be released into your bloodstream. Zinc also helps restore skin cell growth, though it can be irritating if you take it when your stomach is empty.

When you were small, your mother may have given you a few drops of cod liver oil, an important source of vitamins A and D. Today, we know that fish oil can help prevent and heal ulcers because it contains omega-3 fatty acids, which fight inflammation. Beans, nuts, and oil from fish common in northern waters, such as mackerel, salmon and cod, are especially rich in omega-3. You can help protect your gut from ulcers by taking these essential fatty acids in the form of Maxepa supplements, prepared from fish oil.

• *Try Licorice:* This time-honored remedy for ulcers is an ingredient in more than half of Chinese medicine's herbal formulas. Licorice tastes good—it's fifty times sweeter than sugar yet contains no calories —but it has to be used carefully because it can elevate blood pressure. A new product, deglycyrrhizinated licorice (DGL), seems safer because it has eliminated the ingredients that affect blood pressure. In one study, DGL healed ulcers faster than Tagamet or Zantac.

• *Choose Herb Teas and Other Natural Remedies:* Comfrey tea used to be a traditional remedy for ulcers. But because it can become toxic, you should drink it for only a limited period of time. One alternative is slippery elm, a mucilaginous herb that can provide a soothing coating for your stomach lining. Aloe vera is also very healing. Many good cooks keep an aloe vera plant on their kitchen window sill to treat minor burns. When you break off part of a leaf, soothing aloe vera gel oozes out. If you buy aloe vera, make sure you get a gel, its natural form; bottled aloe vera juice is almost all water, sometimes with irritating acidic additives! The young woman with a duodenal ulcer whom I mentioned earlier was given Tagamet and told that her ulcer would heal in three months. On the advice of a nutritionally oriented doctor, she resorted to aloe vera, extra vitamins, and chamomile tea, which soothes spasms and inflammation; her ulcer cleared in six weeks.

Inflammatory Bowel Disease

Inflammatory bowel disease (IBD) is an umbrella term that encompasses two related digestive disorders, Crohn's disease and ulcerative colitis. They affect between one and two million Americans, including one of President Bush's sons, who has ulcerative colitis. Both Crohn's disease and ulcerative colitis involve inflammation of part of your digestive tract. But both chronic diseases are considered systemic: they often are linked to inflammatory disorders in other parts of your body, like arthritis (which troubles a quarter of all IBD patients) or skin problems like psoriasis, eczema, and canker sores in your mouth. IBD, which most often strikes in childhood or young adulthood, can be placed in remission, but it may recur, although years can pass without any symptoms. If left untreated, IBD may have fatal complications, similar to those associated with ulcers. Moreover, there is a higher incidence of colon cancer in people who suffer from ulcerative colitis.

IBD's symptoms, which can range from mild to severe, include fever, excessive gas and bloating, abdominal cramping, rectal itching, pencil- or ribbon-like stools, and frequent bouts of bloody, pus- or mucus-filled diarrhea. IBD sufferers also often have gallstones, kidney stones, and hemorrhoids. A minority of patients with Crohn's disease find blood in their stool; this bleeding can be extremely painful, but also may be consistently painless. People with ulcerative colitis almost always have painful bloody diarrhea at one time or another. A barium x-ray or a colonoscopy, in which the doctor inserts a long, thin, flexible fiberoptic tube into your rectum, will reveal inflammation and perhaps ulceration of your intestinal lining. If you have ulcerative colitis, your colon's lining becomes inflamed and then ulcerated; the ulcers begin to bleed. Inflammation is limited to your colon; your small intestine is not involved. If you have Crohn's disease, the inflammation is likely to be in your small intestine. However, Crohn's disease can affect other parts of your gut, from mouth to anus—hence its common name, regional enteritis, and other names that refer to the part of your intestine that is most affected. Unlike ulcerative colitis, Crohn's disease involves inflammation that deeply penetrates your intestinal wall—sometimes perforating it and spreading to nearby organs like your bladder. If you have either Crohn's disease or ulcerative colitis, you may lose weight and suffer malnutrition.

IBD's symptoms may be ignored because they resemble the flu and milder digestive problems like irritable bowel syndrome. Crohn's disease often announces itself with pain and a lump in your lower right abdomen—symptoms so much like appendicitis that a surgeon might operate before realizing the true nature of your trouble. If you have bloody diarrhea for more than a couple of days, get emergency care right away.

IBD is usually treated with powerful antibiotics, antiinflammatory drugs like sulfasalazine, or with steroids like prednisone. Antibiotics disturb the delicate balance of your friendly intestinal flora, which is extraordinarily complex, made up of over 400 separate microbial species. Because IBD patients may require repeated doses of antibiotics, they risk yeast infections and other intestinal complications. For their part, steroids reduce inflammation and fever, but they are powerful drugs that must be tapered off slowly. Over time, steroids can cause severe side effects, including swelling in your face, hands, and ankles, thinning of your bones and weakening of your joints, and even ulcers, diabetes, cataracts, and psychiatric illness. Moreover, both sulfasalazine and steroids can increase the need for nutrients in patients who have had frequent diarrhea, and who probably are already deficient in vitamins and minerals. Interestingly, Flagyl, an antiparasitic drug, also is often effective in cases of ulcerative colitis. But it does have deleterious side effects, including nausea and malaise, which can be very severe if this drug is ingested with alcohol.

In severe cases, patients may require surgery to remove part or all of their small intestine or colon. Surgery can help Crohn's disease, but rarely cures it: inflammation tends to set in again right next to the part you had removed. Surgery of your colon does cure ulcerative colitis, but has embarrassing cosmetic and psychological aftereffects, as well as important nutritional consequences. Like 23,000 Americans every year, President Bush's third son, Marvin, has had his colon removed, and now has a colostomy: his bodily wastes empty into a pouch through a small tube inserted in his abdomen. At present, he works as a counselor, helping people adjust to living with the consequences of similar surgery. This operation certainly alleviates the considerable distress that IBD causes. But because your intestines are key to absorption of nutrients, surgery is not without long-term nutritional consequences.

LOOKING FOR A CAUSE—AND A SAFE TREATMENT

Medical researchers are still speculating over the cause of IBD. It has been associated with prolonged stress, family history, and Jewish ancestry. Quite a few studies have investigated the possibility that it is an autoimmune disease, the result of an abnormal allergic reaction in which your body's immune system produces antibodies that attack and damage tissue. Some IBD patients have harbored such antibodies, but they appear to be a result of the disease, not its cause. Another possible cause is a virus or bacterium that hasn't been identified yet. Some researchers who embrace this theory think that it is the reason ulcerative colitis sometimes leads to colon cancer.

I think it is important to remember that both ulcerative colitis and Crohn's disease are on the rise in Western countries and are unknown in less developed societies where people eat a great deal of fiber. The high-fat, low-fiber diet that goes with civilization may well be at fault. Several studies have found that those who develop Crohn's disease eat more refined sugar and less raw fruit, vegetables, and dietary fiber than those who remain healthy. One such study found that Crohn's disease patients ate twice as much refined sugar.

There's also a good deal of evidence—more than a dozen studies—implicating food allergies as a contributing factor in the development of IBD in more than half of all cases. Foods most often fingered are wheat, corn, dairy products, citrus fruits, eggs, and sugar. One researcher found that Crohn's disease patients ate cornflakes more frequently. Corn is a common allergen, and cornflakes are high in refined carbohydrates. IBD patients have also found that tomatoes, coffee, bananas, wine, and even tap water may exacerbate their condition.

ONE DOCTOR'S DIET

Dr. De Lamar Gibbons, a general practitioner in Kellogg, Idaho, has suffered from symptoms of IBD since childhood, when he noticed that raisins gave him a skin rash. Gibbons consulted various textbooks, but couldn't find any information linking fructose intolerance to IBD. So he began to monitor the effect that certain foods had on him and his IBD patients. He concluded that an inability to absorb various forms of sugar, especially fructose, is at the root of many IBD cases. The effects of lactose intolerance, he points out, are well documented: if you cannot properly absorb lactose, it ferments into gas, alcohol, and lactic acid, and the result is indigestion. Similarly, Gibbons believes, many people can't turn fructose, sorbitol, or mannitol into glucose. He urges all IBD patients, and arthritis sufferers as well, to read all labels carefully and to rigorously avoid the following:

- All dairy products except yogurt.
- All fruits, honey, maple syrup, and products made with corn syrup. These include soda pop, pastry, candy, cereals, coffee creamers, bottled salad dressings, sweet pickles, cured ham. To detect ubiquitous corn syrup, you must be vigilant about checking ingredients.
- All foods that contain sorbitol or mannitol: sugarless gum and candy, toothpaste, breath mints, processed meats.
- Dr. Gibbons also suggests avoiding hot spices, corn, dried beans, wheat, and wheat bran.

OTHER DRUG-FREE TREATMENTS

- *An Elemental Diet:* Some traditional therapies for colitis have relied on resting your bowel by fasting, drinking only water or vegetable juices. In my experience, this approach is sometimes successful, but can be risky because colitis patients have trouble maintaining weight, and may already be low in nutrients. In their condition, fasting could be nutritionally disastrous, and so it should be undertaken with extreme caution, under the guidance of a competent, nutritionally oriented physician. A safer, but less palatable and more expensive, alternative is to subsist on a food supplement like Vivonex, which is rich in essential nutrients and seldom provokes any allergic reactions. It is even used to nourish AIDS patients, who risk wasting away with chronic diarrhea. But Vivonex has a repulsive taste, even when camouflaged with "flavor packets," and its cost is astronomical. If you do try Vivonex or fasting and these approaches fail, your only alternative is to eat nothing, take appropriate medication, and be fed intravenously.

- *Plenty of Fiber:* Traditionally, most doctors have prescribed little or no fiber for IBD patients, thinking that fibrous foods are too "rough" for their inflamed intestines to handle. Nevertheless, many patients show remarkable improvement on a high-fiber, unrefined-carbohydrate diet. I believe that you should stay away from meat, especially beef. Since many IBD patients are allergic to wheat, psyllium or rice bran may be better choices than wheat bran. Fiber helps whisk out bile acids, which can turn ulcerative colitis into colon cancer.

• *Nutritional Supplements:* Thanks to malabsorption caused by either their disease or their medications, IBD patients usually are low in zinc, magnesium, iron, calcium, potassium, copper, niacin, and vitamins A, B_{12}, C, D, E, and K. They particularly need supplementary folic acid, which keeps inflamed cells from growing in aberrant ways. In this way, folic acid, like vitamin D and calcium, helps reduce the risk of ulcerative colitis becoming colon cancer. Ironically, sulfasalazine, the drug most often prescribed for IBD, depletes folic acid.

• *Butyric Acid:* Like other living things, the cells that line your intestines need sustenance. Their favored nutrient is short-chain fatty acids, especially butyrates. These usually aren't ingested with your meals, but are actually made in your colon. When colonic bacteria break down fiber, butyrates result, and then your intestinal walls absorb them directly. There is some evidence that without butyrates, your colonic mucosa becomes inflamed. In other words, you come down with colitis.

Hence, butyrates are a key part of any program to heal or prevent colitis. They can be taken in supplements or, if dairy products give you no trouble, in goat cheese. Butyric acid is what gives goat cheese its goaty smell.

• *Reduce Inflammation:* Omega-3 fatty acids, in fish oil or in supplements like Maxepa, can help IBD as well as ulcers. So can herbs that fight bacterial overgrowth and herbs known as demulcents, agents that soothe irritated mucous membranes and promote secretion of protective mucus. An ancient herbal remedy known as Bastyr's Formula or Robert's Formula contains several of these herbs, including goldenseal, an antibacterial agent, pokeroot, which soothes inflammation, and slippery elm, a demulcent. Bastyr's Formula also contains cabbage powder to help heal ulcers in your colon.

You may have observed cats or dogs eating grass or even houseplants when they have dyspepsia. They're seeking out chlorophyll, which combats toxins. Taking chlorophyll capsules will help you prevent gastritis and consequently inflammation. They do turn your stool green, but they are particularly useful if you have foul-smelling flatus. N'odor, a form of concentrated chlorophyll, may be a good idea if you have a colostomy and want to minimize odor.

• **Check for Bugs:** Especially if you have been prescribed lengthy courses of antibiotics, you should be tested for a yeast infection and start taking acidophilus supplements and garlic, which helps fight *Candida*. You should also have tests for parasitic infections; your IBD may turn out to be simply an unwanted organism roosting in your gut.

WHAT WE DON'T KNOW ABOUT IBD

Because IBD is still something of a mystery, some researchers and patients have stumbled onto intriguing solutions. For example, Dr. Daniel Present, of New York City's Mount Sinai Hospital, noticed that some smokers develop colitis after they quit. He decided to investigate the benefits of nicotine gum. Although all the evidence isn't in yet, Present says that he has noticed some improvement in colitis patients who chew nicotine gum.

One of my own patients, a young man of about 30, had had intermittently severe colitis since he was 24, requiring several hospital stays, during which he was taken off solid food and fed intravenously to rest his colon. This patient told me that, like many IBD sufferers, he had a relative with the same problem. His grandfather had come down with colitis in his late twenties. Since steroids had not yet been developed, he was told that he was going to die within six months. Figuring he had nothing to lose, he went to a chiropractor, who located and adjusted a pinched nerve. The patient's colitis cleared up. He was so grateful that he named his own son, my patient's father, after the chiropractor. My patient had found that following his grandfather's advice and going to a chiropractor himself, as well as eating plenty of fiber and staying away from sugar, had enabled him to stay off steroids. Conventional medicine might conclude that if chiropractic care made such a difference, grandfather and grandson "obviously did not have colitis." However, poor diet can irritate or overload the neural pathways that go through your spinal cord to various organs, including your colon. While frequently assailed by many practitioners in conventional medicine, chiropractors contend that correcting misalignments in your spine can clear up disorders in various organs, including your digestive tract.

Because having IBD can mean living with severe pain, chiropractic care may help partly because it relieves stress and relaxes you. Some form of stress management or relaxation training also may make a big difference: patients with ulcerative colitis who receive various forms of relaxation training report feeling pain less intensely and less frequently. When pain does strike, they report less emotional upset. If you have IBD, your family and close friends may attend a family therapy or support group to learn how to cope with your problem and help you feel better.

Diverticulosis

No other digestive disease indicts the contemporary American diet as completely as diverticulosis. Dr. Denis P. Burkitt, the prominent British digestive researcher, has called diverticular disease "a deficiency disease of Western civilization" which has become "endemic in our aged citizens."

Today, more than half of all Americans have diverticular disease by the time they turn 60. Burkitt and another researcher, Neil S. Painter, have written, "Diverticular disease was almost unknown in 1900, but has become the commonest affliction of the colon in Western countries within 70 years, the traditional life-span." This dramatic rise in incidence has taken place so quickly that it cannot have a genetic explanation. Moreover, diverticular disease has become so common only in economically developed countries, where diet has changed drastically since the turn of the century. That is when Americans began eating their present diet of refined foods, stripped of most of their fiber. In Africa and Asia, where the diet is still high in fiber, diverticular disease is rare. Painter and Burkitt believe that "the colon's environment has changed," and that diverticular disease is caused by "the diet of so-called civilized countries"—that is, a diet high in meat and refined foods, and low in fiber.

HOW DIVERTICULOSIS STARTS; HOW IT FEELS
Long before you come down with an attack of diverticulitis, you develop diverticulosis, which isn't a disease but a condition of your large intestine that predisposes you to bouts of diverticulitis. When your

colon is healthy, its interior is quite smooth, wavy and undulating. Muscular rings along its length expand and contract up to ten times every minute to move undigested material toward your rectum. Fiber helps this process because it makes your stool moister and bulkier. The softer and more voluminous your stool is, the faster it moves through your colon.

Stools that are low in fiber tend to be drier, and therefore harder and more compact. You become constipated: your colon muscles have to exert more pressure to move your stool. When this happens frequently, as it may if you habitually eat lots of fat and sugar and little fiber, your colon contracts and its walls thicken, particularly in its last section, the sigmoid. This part of your colon is narrower and more muscular, because here your stool is in its most solid form. The added pressure that comes with a thickening of your colon's walls weakens those walls, causing their inner mucosal lining to pop through their outer layers of muscles—pretty much the way an inner tube pokes through a worn rubber tire.

These small pouches are lesions or hernias called diverticula. When you have diverticula, you have diverticulosis. Diverticula can form anywhere in your colon, but are most common in the sigmoid. They make your colon's interior look corrugated, with multiple small folds that you can see clearly in an x-ray photograph. Some researchers think that irritable bowel syndrome (IBS) can contribute to the formation of diverticula. They are not painful or harmful, but they do set the stage for diverticular disease. The diverticula's folds may fill with fecal matter and erode, triggering infection and inflammation. Then you have diverticulitis.

Symptoms of diverticular disease include bloating, nausea, constipation, fever, chills, and sometimes excruciating cramplike pain, especially in your lower left abdomen, near your sigmoid colon. The pain, which may be particularly bad after meals or when you're under stress, can force you into bed. Passing gas or a bowel movement may relieve you, but may also increase your pain. Since these symptoms can indicate other digestive disorders like ulcers, liver disease, or IBS, you will need x-rays to determine whether you have diverticula and whether they are inflamed. If you do have inflamed diverticula, you are in danger of complications. The more dire may occur if your colon's contents burst through holes in your eroded diverticula, spreading infection into your abdomen.

TREATING DIVERTICULITIS

If you have no complications, diverticulitis can clear up after bed rest, a course of antibiotics—which should be complemented by acidophilus supplements to stabilize your intestinal flora—and fasting to rest your colon. You may not need intravenous feeding; three or four days of water or vegetable broth may suffice.

A bout of diverticulitis is a sure sign that you absolutely must change your diet. There is no way that you can smooth out the inside of your colon and rid yourself of diverticula, but you can prevent further attacks of diverticulitis. Besides being painful and potentially dangerous, such attacks ultimately may mean an operation to remove part or all of your diseased colon—surgery that will leave you with a colostomy and an impaired ability to absorb crucial nutrients.

The best way to prevent this unfortunate ending to a case of diverticulitis is to follow the example of Africans and Asians, and switch to a high-fiber diet that is low in sugar and fat. One 1980 study found that by adopting a high-fiber diet, more than 90 percent of patients hospitalized with diverticular disease were able to stay free of symptoms for five to seven years. Although fiber may not cure diverticular disorders, it certainly can reduce or eliminate painful symptoms. For one thing, it makes your stool bulkier, and when your stool is larger, your colon's diameter widens, reducing pressure on diverticula.

THE HOFFMAN DIVERTICULITIS/DIVERTICULOSIS DIET

After the symptoms of diverticulitis have died down, I suggest a week of a soft-fiber diet. Stay away from whole grains and raw vegetables. Sometimes I advise patients to eat only steamed root vegetables, or vegetable soups made in the blender with cooked tomatoes, squash, or peeled cucumbers. You may also eat cantaloupe, watermelon, peeled pears, soaked prunes, olives, tofu, and white rice. You may drink carrot juice or teas made from demulcent herbs like slippery elm, comfrey, and mullein.

For extra bulk to relieve pressure within your colon and to fend off constipation, I recommend a special breakfast of a cleansing herbal mixture of psyllium, bentonite, and myrrh, which is antiinflammatory. Overnight, soak one tablespoonful of this mixture in a cup of water with raisins and prunes. At breakfast the next morning, combine it with grated, peeled apples and pears. I also suggest aloe vera gel, chlorophyll capsules, garlic and acidophilus supplements to help heal your colon and fight harmful bacteria.

Later, patients can eat more soft fiber, like beans, cooked leafy green vegetables, oats, miso, and agar, a form of soluble fiber found in seaweed. At first, it's wise to limit your consumption of whole nuts and seeds, as well as fruits and vegetables with tiny pits or seeds that may stick in diverticula. Some of my patients with diverticular disease have switched to vegetarian or macrobiotic diets. Many who aren't familiar with macrobiotic menus think that you eat nothing but brown rice and beans. Since I've taught classes in macrobiotic gourmet cooking, I can assure you that you can still eat a varied and tasty diet. One patient who embraced macrobiotics, a woman in her sixties, still admits to an occasional weakness for chocolate and croissants. She relies on aloe vera "when I eat the wrong things." Like other patients, this woman also has found that exercise—in her case, in the form of long bicycle rides—has made a big difference in keeping diverticular disease at bay by offsetting constipation.

Gallbladder Disease

The second most common form of abdominal surgery, after cesarean section, is removal of the gallbladder, a small pear-shaped sac located on the right side of your abdomen, below your liver. Your gallbladder concentrates, stores, and then secretes bile from your liver into your small intestine whenever bile is needed to help digest fats. Occasionally a gallbladder attack feels like a mild colic—more of a nuisance than a real pain. An acute attack, however, is marked by very severe pain below your rib cage on the right—some say it is the most excruciating pain you can experience—with vomiting and fever. Such an attack means that your gallbladder is inflamed, usually because of the presence of gallstones.

About 20 million Americans—one tenth of the population—have gallstones, and their ranks swell by another million every year. Gallstones are clumps of solid material, usually crystallized cholesterol, that form in bile when certain chemicals, either cholesterol or bile pigments, start to mass together. Gallstones vary in size; they can be as small as a seed or as big as a golf ball. When stones block the flow of bile from your gallbladder, they cause sharp, constant pain, jaundice (a yellowing of your skin due to backed-up bile), and eventually inflammation.

Gallstones occur more often in people over 60 and in people of Mexican-American or Native American descent. Surgical opinion used to be almost unanimous that gallstones had to be removed. But nowadays, a new consensus holds that only gallstones that provoke chronic symptoms require surgery. The very fact that you have gallstones does not necessarily mean that you must plan a hospital stay. Even if you do have gallstones that are painful right now, some dietary precautions can help you get rid of your symptoms. You may have gallstones for the rest of your life—without their causing you suffering. Here's what you can do to avoid a gallbladder attack and an operation:

• *Lose Extra Weight:* Studies have found that in obese people, bile is supersaturated with cholesterol. This is not true of people whose weight is normal for their height.

• *Stop Crash Dieting:* Losing a great deal of weight quickly seems to contribute to the formation of gallstones. For example, one French study found that women who fast overnight and then skip breakfast the next morning are much more likely to develop gallstones. Even drinking only water for breakfast, researchers noted, would help prevent gallstones.

• *Don't Take Extra Estrogen:* Women who have been pregnant, have used birth control pills, or have had estrogen therapy after menopause are at greater risk of developing gallbladder disease.

• *Stay on a Healthful Diet:* Eating a lot of sugar and not much fiber, especially wheat fiber, can result in gallstones. High dietary cholesterol may be a contributing factor as well. Certainly, a vegetarian diet or the kind of diet that helps prevent heart disease seems to fend off gallstones, too.

• *Check for Food Allergies:* An interesting interpretation of gallbladder attacks links them to allergic reactions to certain foods. In one study, patients with gallstones and symptoms of gallbladder disease found that their symptoms cleared up when they went on a basic elimination diet. The foods most likely to provoke symptoms appeared to be, in descending order, eggs, pork, onions, poultry, milk, coffee, oranges, corn, beans, and nuts. Less frequent food offenders included apples, tomatoes, peas, cabbage, spices, peanuts, fish, rye, and certain medications. Adverse reactions to these foods seem to help form gallstones. Try an elimination diet until your symptoms clear completely.

Then start adding potentially problematic foods, one at a time. You'll soon discover what you can and cannot eat.

TREATING GALLSTONES

Over half a million Americans have their gallbladders removed every year. Although they are able to lead normal lives afterward—you can digest comfortably without a gallbladder—surgery was their only recourse until very recently. In the past, other types of treatment have been limited in their ability to counteract all types of gallstones. Most drugs have had problematic side effects, including diarrhea and liver disease, and are very expensive. However, some new alternatives that work if you have smaller gallstones of a certain consistency seem safer, more effective, and less costly. For some cases, they may make surgery passé except in emergencies.

• *Injection:* The Mayo Clinic, the prestigious medical research center in Rochester, Minnesota, has developed a treatment to dissolve gallstones that involves directly injecting your gallbladder with a form of ether that is usually a gasoline additive. After only a day of ether infusion, painful stones usually disappear—even when they are large or numerous.

• *Shock Waves:* Lithotripsy, a new German technique that uses acoustically generated shock waves, has been used as an outpatient procedure to break up kidney stones painlessly. It is beginning to be used effectively to dissolve gallstones as well. At the moment, lithotripsy requires a trip to the hospital. But you can go home and back to work within a day or two, whereas a gallbladder operation requires a week in the hospital and six weeks of recuperation.

• *Stone-Dissolving Medicine:* Ursodeoxycholic acid, an acid that occurs normally in bile, has been made into a new oral medication, Actigall, to dissolve gallstones made of cholesterol. Complete dissolution takes between one and two years, but stones do recur frequently.

• *High-Tech Surgery:* For uncomplicated cases, pioneering surgical techniques involving minimal incisions can mean that at least some gallstone surgery will require only one day in the hospital. Recently, one of my patients flew to Nashville, Tennessee, for this new laser laparoscopic surgery. After making a small incision, her surgeon used laparoscopy to locate her gallbladder, and then used lasers to excise and remove it. She returned home to New York the next day.

• *Flush Technique:* Finally, there is a natural detoxifying procedure called a liver and gallbladder flush. You administer this procedure yourself at home over the course of a week. Afterward, you may see in your stool the greenish, pea-sized remnants of gallstones. However, a liver flush should be undertaken *only* if you know you have small stones, and *only* under the close supervision of a knowledgeable physician.

OUNCES OF PREVENTION

There are some steps you can take to prevent gallstones as you age or if you become pregnant:

• **Check for Food Allergies:** If you frequently eat any of the foods that may help form gallstones in allergic people, try an elimination diet to spot any adverse reactions.

• **Stick to Vegetables:** A British study has found that the risk of developing gallstones is 1.9 times higher in omnivores than in vegetarians. Staying away from sugar and boosting your fiber intake are helpful, too.

• **Add Fish Oil and Other Nutrients:** There's some evidence that fish oil supplements like Maxepa may protect you from gallstones. People like Greenland's Eskimos, who eat a great deal of fish, have much lower rates of both gallstones and heart disease caused by cholesterol than Americans do. Researchers speculate that fish oil's omega-3 fatty acids may block cholesterol formation in bile. One animal study found that prairie dogs who had a fish oil supplement added to their high-cholesterol diet showed no signs of gallstones. Some other nutrients are helpful, too: lecithin has an emulsifying effect on bile, and taurine, an amino acid, binds to bile salts and speeds their elimination from your body.

• **Drink to Your Health:** Some alcohol intake appears to protect you against gallstones. A 1984 study found that in both sexes, moderate drinkers have fewer gallstones.

Cancer of the Digestive Tract

Unlike some other serious digestive illnesses, cancer is an ancient disease: Hippocrates was the first to identify and describe it. But it occurs far more frequently in modern America than it did in the ancient world. Cancer may develop in any part of your gut, but the most common kind is colon cancer. In fact, after lung cancer, bowel cancer is the most common deadly cancer in America, killing 60,000 people annually.

Every day, roughly 300 new cases of colon cancer come to light. The most obvious warning sign is blood in your stool, which you may not be able to see; it has to be detected by a special test. Other symptoms include abdominal pain, especially after eating, and a change in bowel habits, usually consistently flat or ribbonlike stools and increasing constipation, due to tumorous growth blocking your colon.

Nowadays, when colon cancer is detected early, it can be treated and need not be fatal. Still, you're far better off if you take steps to prevent it from happening to you. Increasingly, the medical establishment's consensus is that cancer often seems to be a disease of overnutrition, its frequency boosted enormously by intake of excess protein, fat, and refined foods like sugar and white flour. Besides smoking, poor diet puts you most at risk for cancer, accounting for up to 70 percent of all cancers. So most of the steps you can take to avoid colorectal and other types of gastrointestinal cancer involve changing your diet.

• **The Fiber Factor:** Colon cancer is still quite rare among people who eat a high-fiber diet. Interestingly, the Japanese had a very low rate of colon cancer until recently, when they began to eat more fast food, refined foods, and other components of the Western diet. On the other hand, in Finland, where people eat even more fat than Americans do, but also ingest considerably more fiber, the rate of colon cancer is one third that of the United States. This suggests that fiber can at least partly counter the harmful effects of dietary fat. Like your stomach, your colon is a part of your gut where your partially digested food remains for a fairly long time. One reason fiber eaters may have cancer less often is that fiber makes your stool bulkier and accelerates transit time, so that any carcinogens you may have eaten along with your meals, as well as potential carcinogens like bile acid, are flushed out of your system rapidly.

Most recently, in 1989, the *Journal of the National Cancer Institute* reported the first direct evidence of fiber's cancer-fighting properties. Researchers found that adding fiber to your diet can prevent precancerous polyps in your colon. Certain kinds of polyps are generally considered precursors of cancer.

• **The Fat Factor:** Fiber also seems to counteract the bad effects of a diet that is high in fat. At this point, there is a great deal of evidence linking fat to cancer: all over the world, a high rate of colon cancer usually follows on the heels of a diet rich in red meat, eggs, and cheese. Lots of fat may stimulate production of lots of bile, which contains cancer-causing chemicals that can irritate and ultimately harm your large intestine's lining.

Certain kinds of fat, however, provide protection against cancer. There is beneficial fat in flaxseed oil and fish oil, which are rich in omega-3 fatty acids. Goat cheese contains butyrate, a short-chain fatty acid that seems to inhibit tumor growth in your colon.

• *The Exercise Factor:* Like fiber, exercise promotes bowel motility, helping to flush carcinogens from your body so that you may avoid colon cancer. A new study, the largest ever carried out to measure fitness, suggests that even modest, not very strenuous exercising can substantially reduce your risk of heart disease, cancer, and other illnesses in both men and women. This means that going from being sedentary to taking a brisk half-hour walk several times a week may help protect you against intestinal cancer.

• *The Calcium Factor:* One reason a high-fiber diet seems to prevent colon cancer is that many fruits and vegetables are high in calcium. Dr. Cedric Garland has spotlighted the roles of calcium and vitamin D, which sunlight helps your body manufacture, in colon cancer prevention. Garland thinks that in your large intestine, calcium combines with bile and harmful fatty acids and whisks them out of your gut. Remember that ingesting excessive amounts of protein and coffee, as well as some types of antacids and laxatives, can impair your body's ability to absorb calcium.

• *The Iron Factor:* Cutting down on protein in the form of red meat is a good idea because too much iron, plentiful in steaks and roast beef, increases your long-term risk for all types of cancer. A new study has found that high stores of iron in your body can set the stage for cancer. Taking iron supplements may be unnecessary or unwise—unless you are pregnant or prone to anemia, and your doctor has advised you to take iron supplements.

• *The Vegetable Factor:* Some researchers think that all vegetables may help prevent cancer. Some surely play a stellar role—carrots, for instance, which are loaded with beta carotene, the plant form of vitamin A. People whose diets are high in beta carotene have lower rates of most types of cancer.

A number of studies have shown that eating cruciferous vegetables —cabbage, broccoli, Brussels sprouts, collards, turnips, and cauliflower—guards against colon cancer. In fact, it may cut your risk by as much as two thirds. A new study in a Chinese province with a very high rate of stomach cancer found that introducing allium vegetables —garlic, scallions, chives, and onions—into the diet reduced rates of illness significantly. The National Cancer Institute has concluded that the more of these vegetables you eat over your lifetime, the lower your chances of developing gastric cancer.

• **The Vitamin C Factor:** Like some other nutrients, including vitamins A and E and selenium, vitamin C helps control and neutralize potentially carcinogenic substances called free radicals, which form in your body through your own metabolism. Certain conditions, including environmental pollution, inflammatory diseases like arthritis, and physiological stress—caused by smoking, poor diet, too much time in the sun, illness, many prescription drugs, or radiation treatments— may increase your production of free radicals and your need for nutrients like vitamin C.

Linus Pauling, who has won Nobel Prizes both for research in chemistry and for peace, has championed megadoses of vitamin C as a healing agent ever since 1970, when he published his popular and controversial book, *Vitamin C and the Common Cold.* In 1978, he and a collaborator, Dr. Ewan Cameron, conducted a study of terminally ill cancer patients, who were each given 10,000 milligrams of vitamin C every day—167 times the United States' Recommended Daily Allowance of 60 milligrams. Pauling and Cameron did not claim that vitamin C cures cancer, but they did note that it ameliorated patients' conditions by generally improving their health and mental outlook. Some patients also lived significantly longer: for example, colon cancer patients lived 142 days longer than average.

Since then, in 1979 and 1985, the Mayo Clinic has responded with two studies that purport to show that vitamin C is no more effective than placebos in slowing cancer or promoting survival. Twice, most recently in 1989, Dr. Pauling has pointed out what he considers flaws in the Mayo Clinic studies, and he continues to maintain that high doses of vitamin C improve the effectiveness of other cancer treatments and prolong the lives of those who are terminally ill.

Aside from Dr. Pauling's work on megadoses of vitamin C, there is some good evidence that ingesting normal amounts reduces the risk of stomach cancer. Almost all cancers are on the rise in America, except for stomach cancer, which has had a dramatic decline. The reason may well be the "citrus revolution"—the fact that citrus fruit and juices are now available all over the country all year long. Stomach cancer seems to be more common in places where people consume very little vitamin C, or less than half the American standard of 60 milligrams daily. You certainly can't lose by eating fresh fruits and vegetables that are rich in vitamin C. The best sources—citrus fruits, tomatoes, green peppers, Brussels sprouts, strawberries, broccoli, cauliflower, fresh leafy green vegetables, cantaloupe, and mangos—are free of fat and full of fiber. If you take your vitamin C in supplements, bear in mind that a single large dose can upset your stomach and give you loose stools. You can avoid these problems by dividing your big doses into two or three smaller doses that you take scattered throughout the day. Buffered vitamin C is also helpful if unbuffered supplements are hard on your gut.

• **The Alcohol Factor:** Most societies with low cancer rates also consume little or no alcohol. Heavy drinking promotes the growth of preexisting cancer cells, causing liver cancer and contributing to cancer of the mouth, throat, and esophagus, especially among smokers.

• **The Yogurt Factor:** There is some evidence that yogurt cultured with *Lactobacillus acidophilus,* and other acidophilus products like kefir and acidophilus milk, can block the activity of an enzyme that can create carcinogens. The University of Nebraska's Dr. Khem Shahani also believes, after many studies, that yogurt made with acidophilus bacteria inhibits tumor growth—good news for all kinds of cancer.

• **The Macrobiotic Factor:** The macrobiotic diet originated in Japan, and grows out of the Oriental medical view of health as balance and disease as imbalance. In principle, the macrobiotic diet is a balanced diet that protects you against degenerative disease. It eliminates meat, dairy products, and sweets and consists of 50 to 60 percent whole cereal grains, 20 to 30 percent fresh vegetables, 5 to 10 percent beans and sea vegetables, and 5 to 10 percent soup made of miso, land or sea vegetables, or fresh fish. You may also eat fresh fruit, nuts, seeds, and fish, depending on where you live and your own needs. An important part of macrobiotic philosophy is eating foods that are in harmony with your environment: for example, depending on the season, you should choose fresh vegetables that are grown locally.

Since the 1960s, the macrobiotic diet has become increasingly popular in this country. According to Michio Kushi, the principal proponent of macrobiotics in America, this diet can help cure cancer. In conventional medicine's view, Kushi's evidence is strictly anecdotal, and the burden is on him and his supporters to come up with hard scientific evidence. Nevertheless, I have personally supervised several patients who, when faced with metastatic colon cancer, have opted for a macrobiotic regimen. Currently, chemotherapy alternatives for this stage of cancer show equivocal benefits at best. Astonishingly, some of these patients are in complete remission today. I also think it is significant that macrobiotic dietary recommendations align with most major government studies and guidelines urging Americans to eat more whole grains, fruits, and vegetables, and to cut down on meat, fat, and sugar.

Staying Well

"Man should always strive to have his intestines relaxed all the days of his life, and that bowel function should approximate diarrhea. This is a fundamental principle in medicine: namely, whenever the stool is withheld or is extruded with difficulty, grave illnesses result."

—Moses ben Maimun (Maimonides),
physician and philosopher, 1135–1204

If you have no chronic digestive problems, minor or serious, I'm delighted. Still, there are some precautions you should start taking in daily life to skirt hazards that could interfere with your good digestion. The principal one, of course, is to stick to a low-fat, high-fiber diet: stay away from sugar, meat, white flour, and other refined foods. Others include keeping an eye out for ubiquitous parasites and maintaining good nutrition under special conditions.

Preventing Food Poisoning

Most foodborne microorganisms that cause illness strike your gastrointestinal tract. Incidence of diseases that can be transmitted by food is rising, even in industrialized nations like the United States. In this country, the Centers for Disease Control document roughly 40,000 cases of food poisoning every year. In reality, according to some estimates, between 20 and 80 million people—up to one third of the population—may suffer food poisoning annually. But millions of cases are overlooked, because people mistake incidents of food poisoning for "that twenty-four-hour bug that's going around." The symptoms, which start within 12 to 48 hours after you eat poisoned food, are similar to flu: nausea, abdominal cramping, diarrhea, fever, headache, and perhaps vomiting. Mild cases pass if you eat a bland diet, drink plenty of water, and allow your illness to run its course. But food poisoning doesn't always pass like a brief bout of flu: perhaps a thousand deaths result every year.

Most people realize that keeping a jar of mayonnaise out of their refrigerator for an extended time is dangerous. But poisonous bacteria have been turning up in foods that no one previously thought could sustain them, partly because more restaurants and cafeterias are relying on precooked foods, and because more people are patronizing salad bars—so that more food stays unrefrigerated for unsafe lengths of time. Some other sources of food poisoning may be overlooked.

• *Chicken:* In 1987, the National Research Council, the research arm of the National Academy of Sciences, reported that about half of the gastrointestinal illness in the United States is caused by poultry contaminated with *Campylobacter jejuni* or *Salmonella* bacteria. According to some estimates, as many as one third to one half of chickens in American markets are contaminated with *Salmonella*, thanks to the way most of them are raised. When birds are reared in cramped quarters and shipped in bulk, fecal matter containing *Salmonella*, which is part of animals' normal intestinal flora, becomes imbedded in their feather follicles and finds its way inside their bodies.

• *Eggs:* The prevalence of *Salmonella* has affected eggs as well: since 1979, the incidence of salmonellosis from eating grade A eggs has increased sixfold in New England, and is spreading to other parts of the country. Foods that contain raw or undercooked eggs, like homemade eggnog or Caesar salad dressing, have also caused cases of salmonellosis. The bacteria have even cropped up in egg products like pasta.

• *Dairy Products:* In 1985, more than 16,000 cases of salmonellosis, including four deaths, were confirmed after raw milk in an Illinois dairy plant leaked into a tank of pasteurized milk. Other dairy products, including cheese and chocolate, have caused *Salmonella* poisoning.

• *Red Meat and Antibiotics:* A particularly disturbing development has been the appearance of strains of *Salmonella* that resist antibiotics. In 1987, researchers found that people recently treated with antibiotics, especially tetracycline, one of four antibiotics most often prescribed, had a significantly greater risk of becoming infected with resistant strains of *Salmonella*. Taking antibiotics may make you more vulnerable because your medication strips your large intestine of its beneficial flora, leaving you more susceptible to *Salmonella*.

One probable reason for the growth in resistant *Salmonella* strains is the widespread use of antibiotics in farm-animal feed to promote growth and prevent illness in cows and pigs. According to the Federal Drug Administration, more than 40 percent of antibiotics produced in this country are fed to animals being reared for food. As much as 80 percent of pork and 66 percent of beef sold in the United States come from animals who have been fed antibiotics.

• *Fish and Shellfish:* Raw fish and shellfish are frequently culprits in cases of food poisoning caused by viral or bacterial infection. If you are fond of sushi, steer clear of homemade varieties; enjoy it only in reputable Japanese restaurants where chefs are especially trained to select and prepare clean, disease-free fish. Fish from waters contaminated with sewage or other waste may carry bacteria and viruses on their bodies or in their guts. Their flesh is usually clean, but you could be infected if you cut your hands while cleaning them or handling fish hooks.

And if you favor clams and oysters, try to avoid eating them raw. In 1982, outbreaks of gastroenteritis due to eating raw shellfish infected with a viral strain reached epidemic proportions in New York State. Shellfish may also transmit dangerous hepatitis A, and thanks to illegal harvesting from contaminated areas, infected clams and oysters are more likely to turn up on your plate.

HOW TO PREVENT GASTRONOMIC DISASTER

According to estimates from the Centers for Disease Control, over two thirds of cases of food poisoning are due to food served outside the home, and about 5 percent can be blamed on commercially prepared food. Be cautious when you eat out: while you certainly can order sushi in a good restaurant, you're better off avoiding rare or uncooked meat delicacies like steak tartare. And if you aren't planning to eat your take-out salad or sandwich right away, refrigerate it promptly.

But over a quarter of cases of food poisoning happen thanks to home cooking! Here are some steps you can take to protect yourself and your family.

• *To Be Safe, Refrigerate:* Keep your freezer at zero degrees Fahrenheit or lower, and your refrigerator below 40 degrees Fahrenheit; at higher temperatures, *Salmonella* thrives in meat, poultry, dairy products, and eggs. Temperatures normally reached during boiling, baking, frying, and roasting usually destroy *Salmonella*. Use your refrigerator to thaw or marinate food—not your kitchen counter. Contrary to widespread popular belief, eggs, butter, and cooked vegetables do need immediate and constant refrigeration. Never leave raw or cooked food out of your refrigerator for more than two hours.

• *Wash Up:* Wash meat, fish, poultry, and raw vegetables thoroughly. Wash your hands before cleaning fish or cutting up meat, and don't lick your fingers or utensils while you're working. Wash your hands again, along with utensils, cutting boards and counters, after contact with raw meat, eggs, fish, or poultry. Don't place cooked meat, fish, or poultry on plates that have held raw fish, fowl, or meat. Even though cooking kills most microorganisms that cause gastrointestinal illness, your food can easily become recontaminated if it touches raw food or surfaces or utensils that are still contaminated.

• *Shop Carefully:* If you want to eat raw meat or eggs at home, buy organic products from free-range animals—chickens, beef cattle, and pigs raised without antibiotics, in pens away from other animals, where they have room to move about freely. Free-range meat and eggs cost more, but they are far more likely to be free of *Salmonella*. Never buy or use cracked raw eggs. Ask your butcher to stock meat from suppliers who don't use antibiotics in animal feed, and as much as you can, avoid taking unnecessary antibiotics.

• *Cook Thoroughly:* Cook chicken until there are no pink juices running from the joints, the parts that cook most slowly. Cook pork until the pink is gone, fish until it flakes. Rare, undercooked beef is safe provided you eat it within a half hour of cooking. Turn microwaved foods, and check for uneven cooking. If you go on a summer picnic, be aware that ice will preserve your meal only until it melts. Refrigerate leftovers right away, and if you aren't going to use them promptly, freeze them.

Tips for Travelers

Collectively, Americans spend more than the gross national product annually on travel. Unfortunately, that means that more Americans are returning home with gastrointestinal symptoms. By far the most common is acute diarrhea. If your problem is "Montezuma's revenge" or traveler's diarrhea, thanks to eating or drinking something contaminated with a harmful bacterial strain like *E. coli, Salmonella,* or *Campylobacter,* your illness will run its course, and your health will improve once you're home. But if you have picked up a parasite, like *Giardia lamblia* or *Entamoeba histolytica,* your diarrhea will persist, and may even be bloody. Your other symptoms can include bloating, gas, abdominal pain, anal itching, and even fever, chills, severe fatigue, and skin rashes. You may even show signs of malabsorption and what appear to be food allergies.

Diagnosing parasitic infections often takes a long time, because their symptoms may be mistaken for irritable bowel syndrome and other digestive disorders. And treatment can be difficult and prolonged. One course of a single drug may not rid you completely of a parasite—and you may be infected with more than one variety. Some patients with amebiasis have to take Flagyl, which, if you consume it with alcohol, can make you as ill as if you'd taken Antabuse.

Traveler's diarrhea and parasitic infections used to be associated with trips to remote, underdeveloped countries. But nowadays, the spread of some organisms, combined with lax enforcement of standards for public drinking water, means that you can come down with traveler's diarrhea in the United States or pick up a parasite in Europe. Depending on where you're going, it may be hard to protect yourself completely, but here are some pointers.

DODGING "THE RUNS"

Traveler's diarrhea can be very difficult to avoid, no matter how cautious you are. One of my patients traveled extensively in the mountains of eastern Mexico, staying in remote inns. She was never ill until she checked into a major tourist hotel in Mexico City—and ordered room service. *Salmonella* can lurk in airline food and in canapés on cruise ships, as well as in exotic treats like Kenyan cashew nuts, Thai smoked salmon, Indonesian raw prawns, Taiwanese shrimp, and Malaysian black pepper. In many places, however, the major hazard is water. So standard precautions against traveler's diarrhea include drinking only commercially bottled and sealed water, or water that has been boiled or treated. Use bottled water to brush your teeth. Hot coffee and tea, beer, liquor, wine and carbonated beverages are safe, provided you don't use ice.

In many countries, water used to grow and wash foods is contaminated with sewage or is poorly purified. If you eat fresh fruits or vegetables, pick ones you can peel yourself, like bananas or cucumbers. Cooked vegetables should be safe. Avoid buying fresh or prepared foods at open-air markets or from street vendors, no matter how tempting or colorful.

In some parts of the world, including Africa, Malta, Spain, and Australia, dairy products may be unpasteurized and apt to contain bacteria that cause brucellosis, a potentially severe infection. When in doubt, your best bet is to rely on powdered milk mixed with boiled water.

To help combat traveler's diarrhea, many doctors used to recommend prophylactic doses of antibiotics, which you were supposed to start taking before you left home. But because antibiotics upset the delicate balance of your friendly intestinal flora, they are apt to provoke gastrointestinal symptoms instead of preventing them. Moreover, travelers who routinely take antacids to offset indigestion after exotic foreign cuisine are more at risk of bacterial infection because these medications suppress your stomach's production of hydrochloric acid, which normally furnishes you with powerful protection against unfriendly microorganisms. Here is just one striking example from medical history: in the 1850s, a researcher named Max von Pettenkofer swallowed a hefty portion of cholera bacillus. Surprisingly, nothing happened to him—and he claimed that he had disproved Robert Koch's theory that bacteria cause illness. However, Pettenkofer's critics retorted that his stomach was producing an excessive amount of gastric acid at the time—enough to safeguard him even from cholera.

One over-the-counter remedy that does seem to ward off traveler's diarrhea without harmful gastrointestinal side effects is Pepto-Bismol. Its main ingredient, bismuth, prevents traveler's diarrhea in about 65 percent of people who take two chewable tablets (much easier to pack than bottles of pink liquid) four times daily. Once traveler's diarrhea hits, chewing one tablet every hour can help bring your bowel movements back to normal.

According to Daniel Gagnon, a Santa Fe, New Mexico, herbalist, acidophilus capsules can also help fend off traveler's diarrhea. Start taking a couple a day two weeks before you leave on your trip, and continue to take them while you're away. Moderate amounts of coffee, tea, and hot spices all stimulate your stomach's production of hydrochloric acid, so choose your menu accordingly while you're on the road.

PREVENTING PARASITES

Amebiasis is still a scourge outside the United States. In poorer countries, according to the World Health Organization, one in ten people is apt to be infected. Worldwide, amebiasis kills up to 100,000 every year. However, in the United States and in parts of western and eastern Europe, infection with the *Giardia* parasite, also known as "beaver fever," qualifies as an epidemic. *Perestroika* notwithstanding, if you are traveling to Leningrad, the U.S. State Department warns you not to drink the tap water there, which is contaminated with *Giardia*.

Giardia, an elusive and ubiquitous bug, spreads when beavers defecate into mountain streams. Consequently, outbreaks of *Giardia* infection have been reported in chic mountain resorts like Aspen, Colorado. From mountain streams, *Giardia* finds its way into municipal water supplies. Chlorination does not eradicate this hardy microorganism, so unless your water supply is also filtered, *Giardia* may turn up in public drinking fountains and your own tap water.

In this country, travelers most at risk of *Giardia* infection are backpackers, mountain climbers, and hikers who may be tempted to drink from seemingly pristine woodland lakes and brooks. However, according to the National Park Service, you should assume that *Giardia* is present in all natural water, no matter how remote it is from civilization, how cold the water is, how rapidly it runs, or how close you are to the source of a brook or spring. Many campers carry chlorine and iodine tablets to purify water, but these are neither very good for you nor strong enough to purge *Giardia*. The best protection is a lightweight, portable water filtering system, which any camper or backpacker can carry easily.

If you are a traveler who isn't camping out, but who wants to guard against *Giardia* and other parasites, take the same precautions with local water and raw fruit and vegetables as you would to avoid traveler's diarrhea. Eat cooked food while it is still hot. Insist on being served meat that is well done: pig roasts in Oceania or steak tartare in Paris may leave you vulnerable to parasitic or bacterial infection. You're better off if you pass up raw fish and shellfish: some experts believe that sushi restaurants may be safer in the United States than in Japan or other parts of Asia. In the Netherlands, Scandinavia, and the Orient, parasites ingested with raw herring or sushi have caused gastrointestinal symptoms resembling those of Crohn's disease or acute appendicitis.

Some parasites can penetrate your skin. Especially in Third World countries, try to avoid swimming in fresh water. Salt water is generally free of parasites, although it may be contaminated with sewage. Avoid strolling barefoot on beaches.

Rather than taking antibiotics as prophylaxis against parasites, take four capsules of garlic three times a day. Garlic's antibacterial properties are well documented, and it may also be effective against parasites. Artemisia (also known as wormwood), kelp, plums, and jalapa leaves, grown in Mexico, are other traditional remedies. Daniel Gagnon also recommends taking digestive bitters and ten drops of Ileocecal Tonic before each meal while traveling. He takes echinacea to boost his immune system and ward off jet lag.

If you are diagnosed with a *Giardia* infection, you are probably suffering from malabsorption, and consequently may be undernourished. Bear in mind that besides taking prescribed medications, eating plenty of protein and taking vitamin and mineral supplements are an important part of your recovery.

MOTION WITHOUT AGONY
If you are plagued by motion sickness, traveling by plane, automobile or boat may be nightmarish. Ginger capsules can be helpful, and so can acupressure wrist bands, tight bracelets that bear down on a spot near your wrist, relaying nerve impulses to the vertigo center in your brain. These bracelets are available from Travel Accessories, P.O. Box 391162, Solon, Ohio 44139, (216) 248-8432.

Caring for Children

The first gastrointestinal disorder you associate with children may be your own morning sickness during pregnancy. Ginger and acupressure bracelets, the solutions for motion sickness, may make a difference. Raspberry leaf tea is another time-honored remedy.

When babies are born, their guts are sterile. Once they start to eat, however, gastrointestinal trouble may set in. At the turn of the century, about half of all American babies were breast-fed for at least the first year of their lives. By the 1970s, about one in three babies was breast-fed during the first month of life. Today, while breast-feeding is becoming more popular, only about 5 percent of infants nurse until they are six months old, and only 1 percent nurse throughout their first year.

In this country, part of the reason more babies aren't breast-fed is that many mothers assume that "milk is milk," and that whether a newborn drinks mother's milk or cow's milk makes no big difference. Many people also assume that thanks to modern technological expertise, artificial infant formulas can duplicate the quality of mother's milk. Both of these assumptions are myths.

Indeed, many differences between cow's milk and human milk have been minimized in modern infant formulas. But babies do absorb some nutrients better, including iron and zinc, if they ingest them in breast milk. Most important, colostrum, the milklike substance that precedes the flow of milk from a mother's breast, and human milk itself both provide newborns with antibodies and beneficial flora that colonize their intestines. Premature infants who subsist on formula, and who frequently are given large doses of antibiotics to help them survive, are often prey to gastrointestinal infections because they do without breast milk. Some studies have found that babies fed breast milk alone, as opposed to a combination of mother's milk and cow's milk, have far fewer gastrointestinal infections, and respiratory infections as well. In another study, infants fed formula alone had six times more gastrointestinal illness than those given breast milk alone, and two and a half times more illness than babies fed cow's milk only. Small amounts of human milk can kill parasitic protozoa like *Giardia lamblia* and *Entamoeba histolytica*, both of which can cause acute gastrointestinal illness.

If you breast-feed, however, what you ingest eventually reaches your baby. Nursing mothers who have one or more alcoholic drinks daily may pass along enough alcohol in their milk to slightly retard their infants' motor development. Then their babies may learn to crawl and walk more slowly. Nursing mothers also cannot take certain drugs because they affect either milk production or infants themselves. If you are obliged to take medication, consult with your doctor to find out if drug therapy is absolutely necessary, and which is the safest type of drug to take.

Once you stop nursing, there is always a possibility that your baby cannot tolerate cow's milk. Very few infants have lactose intolerance, but inability to tolerate cow's milk is quite common. Many newborns suffer from colic: they alternate between general fussiness and agonized crying, especially late in the day. They clench their fists, draw up their legs, and scrunch up their faces in pain. Their main problem seems to be excess gas; burping may relieve them, but only temporarily. Some researchers think that colic is an infant variation of irritable bowel syndrome, which may be remarkably frequent in children as well as in adults. The culprit may be cow's milk. Suffering babies also may have frequent diarrhea, or alternate between diarrhea and constipation. If your baby cannot tolerate cow's milk, you may have to switch to a soybean or other formula.

Sometimes babies who are being breast-fed or given cow's milk have severe, bloody diarrhea. This can be a sign that they cannot tolerate protein in cow's milk. Even breast-fed babies may suffer if their mothers are drinking cow's milk while they are nursing. Once their mothers stop drinking milk, infants' symptoms pass. Some babies who are particularly allergic cannot even tolerate protein in soybean formula.

AS BABIES GROW

Unfortunately, some soybean formulas and other baby foods are sweetened with corn syrup, and so some babies may be colicky because they cannot tolerate fructose. Some studies indicate that small children have a limited ability to absorb fructose. Apple juice, whose sugar content is largely in the form of fructose, can cause babies abdominal pain, diarrhea, and malabsorption. Try eliminating apple juice, and see if your baby's diarrhea passes. Another ingredient that may give infants diarrhea is sorbitol. Both apple and pear juice are high in sorbitol. If you suspect that your baby's trouble is sorbitol intolerance, try grape juice, which contains no sorbitol.

Early in 1989, many parents became concerned about apples and apple juice after the Natural Resources Defense Council, a private environmental group, publicized the fact that many apple growers spray their crops with a potentially dangerous pesticide, Alar. According to the NRDC, children's sensitivity and possible exposure to pesticides in food is six to twelve times greater than that for adults, who generally ingest fewer fruits and vegetables. Rather than shopping for prepared baby foods and beverages, some parents are buying organic produce and using juicers or food mills to make baby food that they are certain is free of chemicals and full of nutrients.

As children grow, they become increasingly tempted by fast food and junk food. Researchers who are interested in encouraging changes in the Western diet to prevent digestive disease have noted that the single most important factor influencing what people choose to eat is social custom. Since social pressure begins at home, you can set your children a good example by sticking to a healthful diet yourself. Dr. Herbert M. Shelton, the father of food combining, wrote, "It is vitally important that growing children have a daily salad. Indeed, the salad is more important for the growing child than for the adult, although it is very important for the adult. Children should be started early in life with their daily salad so that they build a keen relish for it and continue to eat it for the rest of their lives. . . . These salads are more acceptable sources of calcium than is milk"—and quite safe if your child cannot tolerate lactose.

If You're Very Active

An exercise program can contribute significantly to preventing digestive problems, especially constipation. Because exercise relaxes you, it offsets the deleterious effects that stress may have on your gut. Some exercises, especially tennis, rowing, and other sports that tone your abdomen, can contribute to good digestion. If you tend to have heartburn or irritable bowel syndrome, extended runs, especially right after a meal, can bring on "runner's reflux." If you run early in the morning, don't have a cup of coffee before you set out; it will increase reflux.

If you're particularly athletic, you especially need a nutritious diet. Until very recently, athletes were thought to need mostly complex carbohydrates—found in whole grains, potatoes, beans, fresh fruits and vegetables—rather than a high-protein diet. It is certainly possible to be a vegetarian athlete, and some major competitors are. But new findings indicate that athletes do need more protein, so choose yours from lean sources like fish and poultry, or from combined vegetarian sources, like beans and rice or whole wheat bread with peanut butter. Since dehydration is always a risk for athletes, make sure you drink plenty of water, your most important nutrient.

Strenuous physical activity may mean that your need for certain nutrients, including several B vitamins, vitamins C and E, and some minerals, is higher than the Recommended Daily Allowance. Bear in mind, however, that while you may need supplements, they will not give you energy. They simply help you augment a healthful diet so that you will have that competitive edge when you need it most.

If You're Over 65

Older people are more at risk for every digestive disease and disorder, especially colon cancer and diverticulosis and diverticulitis, which generally develop after the age of 40. They often are reaping the dubious rewards of a lifetime on a high-fat, low-fiber diet. Poor nutrition probably ages you more rapidly and contributes to higher rates of illness and early death.

For several reasons, the elderly also are more likely to suffer malabsorption and therefore deficiencies of vital nutrients. Elderly people use more medications than any other group in America; the average person over 65 takes two medications every day, either for chronic illnesses or for minor complaints. Because many drugs cause malabsorption or mineral depletion, they compound the risk of malnutrition in elderly people.

As your gut ages, your stomach secretes less hydrochloric acid, so that you have trouble absorbing some nutrients, including iron. Because "acid stomach" is a frequent harbinger of aging, many older people compound their problem by relying heavily on antacids. These medications suppress your stomach's production of hydrochloric acid, leaving you more at risk for gastrointestinal illness caused by parasitic, bacterial, or viral infection. Antacids can even contribute to indigestion, because sooner or later, your stomach rebounds, pouring out even more hydrochloric acid. Many elderly people also have a habit of using laxatives, especially if they are unused to combatting constipation by exercising and eating fiber. Mineral oil, a common laxative ingredient, increases your body's excretion of fat-soluble vitamins. If you suffer from night blindness, check the label on your laxative; mineral oil may be depleting you of fat-soluble vitamin A.

If you have osteoporosis, a brittleness of the bones which plagues as many as 80 percent of women over 65, your laxative also may be part of the problem because you are losing fat-soluble vitamin D, which strengthens your bones. Bone-thinning is a consequence of aging which begins when you are in your thirties. Your risk of osteoporosis is higher if you have had gastroplasty, surgery which used to be performed for obesity. Osteoporosis can be exacerbated by lack of exercise and a diet that is low in calcium and vitamin D. The best sources of calcium are fresh vegetables and fruit, which are also high in fiber. If you are over 40, taking calcium supplements is a good preventive measure. Some women regularly take Tums, a popular over-the-counter antacid, because it is also a source of calcium. But Tums can cause constipation as well as other side effects associated with antacids. The best available form of calcium supplements is calcium citrate, which is not constipating.

To Conclude . . .

The number and severity of digestion-related problems that you may incur as you grow older can be quite chilling to contemplate. In old age, after years of poor diet compounded by multiple medications, digestion frequently is so problematic that it is many older people's principal concern—even obsession. Fortunately, it is never too late to make a change for the better—to opt for a healthier diet and eating habits. Even if you have no digestive trouble at all today, consider whether your present habits are putting you in danger of discomfort and even disease later on in life. Like every other part of you, your gut ages. When you are younger, your gastrointestinal tract may be resilient enough to bounce back from repeated mistreatment. But eventually, those chickens you ate—or more likely, those hamburgers, hot dogs, ice cream cones, and cans of soda and beer—will come home to roost in your troubled gullet.

You can't dodge the fact that you are what you eat. Rabelais describes a character who tries—a queen whose attendants faithfully chewed her food for her, poured it into her stomach through a gold funnel, and even "sat on the close-stool by proxy"! Of course, this queen could do all this for herself—but thank heavens, she didn't have to! It's too bad this approach isn't available to all of us; digestive disease might become obsolete. Instead, you have to opt for preventive measures. Even if you are pain-free today, take the Hoffman Program seriously: it will save you trouble and medical costs tomorrow.

And if you are in pain, remember—*you don't have to live with it.* After one of my patients, Louise, a tall slender woman in her early fifties, suffered three very painful attacks of diverticulitis in 1983, she made the rounds of several doctors. "I thought I was eating pretty sensibly," she recalls. "I certainly never overate. I couldn't imagine what was wrong with me. I asked to see my x-rays, and it was the biggest shock to find those diverticula that had formed in my colon." By the time Louise consulted me, she had tried fasting and antibiotics, neither of which seemed to stave off her recurring pain. Other doctors had been telling her she ought to "think about an operation."

When I began to take Louise's medical history, I discovered that she had grown up in France, and that her mother, now in her eighties, also had diverticulosis. Not surprisingly, given her gastronomic heritage, Louise was fond of croissants, chocolate, cheese, and other rich, creamy dairy products. I put Louise on my Diverticulosis Diet, encouraging her to eat only steamed vegetables for the first week—a regimen with plenty of soft fiber that would not abrade her damaged colon. I also suggested that she take acidophilus and chlorophyll capsules every day to prevent pathogenic bacteria from gaining the upper hand again, along with emulsifying herbs like slippery elm bark and healing aloe vera.

Louise took her illness for what it was—a sign that she was obliged to change her eating habits. Like a true Frenchwoman, she took eating and its pleasures very seriously. Recognizing that old habits die hard, she took a series of classes in gourmet vegetarian and macrobiotic cooking, so that her new diet would be as tempting as possible. These courses taught her that reorganizing her diet would take time and effort. So she even restructured her life, switching from a very stressful job as a secretary in television production to doing accounting for a real estate firm, where her hours were flexible and her bosses less demanding. Best of all, she could work at home or bring her own meals to her office, so that she was able to eat exactly as she wanted. Finally, she abandoned her sedentary way of life and took up bicycling.

Louise has been faithful to her new habits, and today, she has been free of pain for several years. She confesses that every now and again, she indulges in a croissant or a piece of chocolate, quickly followed by a dose of aloe vera to avoid painful consequences. My main point, however, is that she has reduced a *steady* intake of fats and sugar to an occasional treat. And she's genuinely not tempted to stray far from a better way of eating, because she's made her meals so delectable. Instead of spending her vacations with relatives in France, going from one rich meal to another, she takes group bike trips, bringing much of her food with her.

Like Louise, you may not immediately find a magic formula that will clear up your digestive pain. Especially if you turn out to have a parasitic infection, you may need a series of tests and more than one type of treatment to eradicate your problem. You—and your doctor as well—may have to summon up patience, fortitude, and a fair amount of ingenuity. But keep in mind that, as Louise found out, eating better doesn't have to mean saying goodbye to all the pleasure you're used to having at mealtime. Instead, by cultivating new tastes, you can have a good time without having to pay a horrendous price in pain and poor digestion. To your health!

Sources

CHAPTER ONE

Tagamet's history is described in "Companies Search for Next $1 Billion Drug," by Gina Kolata, *The New York Times*, November 28, 1988. Zantac's success is reported in "SmithKline, Beecham to Merge," by Steve Lohr, *The New York Times*, April 13, 1989. The Public Citizens Health Research Group's *Over the Counter Pills That Don't Work* (New York: Pantheon, 1983) details the shortcomings of antacids and other over-the-counter remedies for stomach pain. The National Commission on Digestive Diseases 1978 Report to the U.S. Congress documents the incidence of and expenses related to digestive problems. The July 1988 issue of the *American Journal of Clinical Nutrition* documents the way medical education frequently neglects training in nutrition. The results of the second National Health and Nutrition Examination Survey (NHANES II) are analyzed by Block et al. in "Nutrient Sources in the American Diet: Quantitative Data from the NHANES II Survey" in the *American Journal of Epidemiology* 1985; 122:27–40. Marshall Efron makes a lemon pie in the film "A Chemical Feast," distributed by Benchmark Films, Inc. *The Paleolithic Prescription*, by S. Boyd Eaton, M.D., Marjorie Shostak, and Melvin Konner, M.D., Ph.D. (New York: Harper & Row, 1988) describes the caveman diet. A reasonable facsimile is endorsed by the National Research Council's report *Diet and Health* (Washington,

D.C.: National Academy Press, 1989). Statistics on the number of prescriptions some specialists write every week for certain drugs are drawn from the July 1988 Media-Chek from the International Medical News Group in New York. Much of "A Brief History of Bran" is drawn from "ABC of Nutrition," by A. Stewart Truswell, *British Medical Journal* 1985; 291:1486–90, and "History of Promotion of Vegetable Cereal Diets," by Daphne A. Roe, *Journal of Nutrition* 1986; 116:1355–63.

CHAPTER TWO

William Hunter's opinion appears in F. Gonzalez-Crussi's essay on the "Rapunzel Syndrome" in *Notes of an Anatomist* (San Diego, California: Harcourt Brace Jovanovich, Inc., 1985). Dr. William Beaumont's and Ivan Pavlov's experiments, along with the general workings of the digestive system, are well described in *Reader's Digest ABC's of the Human Body* (Pleasantville, New York: Reader's Digest Association, 1987) and Isaac Asimov's *The Human Body: Its Structure and Operation* (Boston: Houghton Mifflin, 1963). These books are also the major sources of the figures and anatomical locations in the two sidebars accompanying this chapter. A discussion of satiety and the link between the brain and the gut appears in "Brain-Gut Peptides and Postprandial Satiety," a paper presented at the 1989 meeting of the American Association for the Advancement of Science by Nori Geary, Department of Psychology, Columbia University. One study of the importance of thorough chewing to good digestion is "Oral Digestion of a Complex-Carbohydrate Cereal: Effects of Stress and Relaxation on Physiological and Salivary Measures," by Donald R. Morse et al., *American Journal of Clinical Nutrition* 1989; 49:97–105. The father of food combining, Herbert M. Shelton, explained his ideas in *Food Combining Made Easy* (San Antonio, Texas: Willow Publishing, 1982). The principles of food combining are also the basis of the "Fit for Life" diet described in *Fit for Life*, by Harvey Diamond and Marilyn Diamond (New York: Warner Books, 1985). The idea of a second "brain" in the gut is described in "The Stomach's Link to the Brain," by Stewart Wolf, *Federation Proceedings* 44; 14:2889–93, November 1985. The pioneering researchers who first discussed the role of fiber in speeding toxins and pathogens out of the body are Denis P. Burkitt and Hugh C. Trowell, in *Refined Carbohydrate Foods and Disease: Some Implications of Dietary Fibre* (London and New York: Academic Press, 1975). The idea that happiness promotes good digestion is a precept of shiatsu expert Wataru Ohashi, director and principal instructor of the Ohashi Institute and author of *Do-It-Yourself Shiatsu* (New York: E. P. Dutton, 1976). The number of Americans who suffer heartburn is documented in the Gallup Organization survey "Heartburn Across America," sponsored by Glaxo, Inc. William T. Parker et al. discuss some of the effects of intestinal bypass surgery in the *American Journal of Gastroenterology* 1985; 80:535–37. Dr. George Crile's opinion on treating appendicitis appears in *Dissent in Medicine: Nine Doctors Speak Out* (Chicago: Contemporary Books, 1985). Dr. Cedric Garland and Dr. Frank Garland describe the roles of calcium and fiber in preventing colon cancer in *The Calcium Connection*, which they wrote with Ellen Thro (New York: Simon and Schuster, 1989).

CHAPTER THREE

Smoking

An excellent fact sheet on *Smoking and Your Digestive System*, by James Walter Kikendall, M.D., and Lawrence F. Johnson, M.D. (NIH Publication No. 87–949) is available free of charge from National Digestive Diseases Education and Information Clearinghouse, Box NDDIC, Bethesda, Maryland 20892, (301)469-6344. Some of the studies linking smoking and digestive cancer include P. Mills et al., "Dietary Habits and Past Medical History as Related to Fatal Pancreas Risk Among Adventists," *Cancer* 1988; 61:2578–85; Harry Daniell, "More Advanced Colonic Cancer Among Smokers," *Cancer*, 1986; 58:784; studies by Dr. Neal L. Benowitz et al. at the University of California at San Francisco ("Nicotine Absorption and Cardiovascular Effects with Smokeless Tobacco Use: Comparison with Cigarettes and Nicotine Gum," *Clinical Pharmacology and Therapeutics* 44; 1:23–28, July 1988; "Daily Use of Smokeless Tobacco: Systemic Effects," *Annals of Internal Medicine* 1989; 111:112–16) found that tobacco chewers face abnormally high risks of developing cancers of the digestive system from absorbing large quantities of nicotine through saliva and mouth tissue. A 1988 study by Dr. Richard Hurt et al. at the Mayo Clinic's Smoking Cessation Center was reported in "77% in Study of Nicotine Patch

Quit Smoking," *The New York Times*, April 30, 1989. The rise of caffeine levels in the blood of people who quit smoking but continue to drink the same amount of coffee was documented by Dr. Neal L. Benowitz et al. at San Francisco General Hospital and reported in *The British Medical Journal*, July 1989. The effect of smoking on smokers' weight and waist-to-hip ratio is part of the 26-year Baltimore Longitudinal Study of Aging at the National Institute on Aging, led by Reubin Andres, M.D., et al.

Caffeine

The popularity of coffee and tea is documented by Gladys Block et al. in "Nutrient Sources in the American Diet: Quantitative Data from the NHANES II Survey," *American Journal of Epidemiology* 1985; 122:27–40. This study is also the basis of the information in the sidebar "America's Eating Habits: Expressway to a Stomachache." Most of the information in the sidebar "Hidden Caffeine" was compiled by the Institute of Food Technologists from various industry and government sources, and published in Jane E. Brody's "Personal Health" column in *The New York Times*, May 18, 1989. The effects of caffeine on excretion of nutrients are documented by L. Massey and P. Hollingbery in "Acute Effects of Dietary Caffeine and Aspirin on Urinary Mineral Extraction in Pre- and Postmenopausal Women," *Nutrition Research* 1988; 8:845–51. Caffeine's effect on the gastrointestinal tract is discussed in *Food Allergy and Intolerance*, by Jonathan Brostoff and Stephen J. Challacombe (Eastbourne, England: Buillière Tindall, 1987). Several studies have documented the effect of coffee and decaf on cholesterol level; among the most recent is the work of Dr. H. Robert Superko at the Stanford Lipid Research Clinic, published in the *Medical Journal of Circulation* (vol. 80, October 1989) and reported in *The New York Times*, November 15, 1989 ("Decaffeinated Coffee Tied to Cholesterol Rise") and November 23, 1989 ("Study Finds Boiled Coffee Raises Cholesterol"). At the Bowman Gray School of Medicine, Drs. Donald O. Castell, Daniel W. Murphy, and W. C. Wu have documented that chocolate exacerbates heartburn in *Internal Medicine News* 20; 15:3. Dr. Judith Wurtman, a cellular biologist at the Massachusetts Institute of Technology, describes her findings on sugar and seratonin in her book *Managing Your Mind and Mood Through Food* (New York: Rawson Associates, 1986).

Alcohol

Many studies have documented the deleterious effects of alcohol on nutrition and digestion. Most of the information in this section came from the National Institutes of Health and the October 1987 issue of *Nutrition and the M.D.*, vol. 13, no. 10. The survey of French drinking habits was conducted by the weekly *Le Nouvel Observateur* and reported in *The New York Times*, December 7, 1988.

Sugar

The exhibition "The Confectioner's Art" was organized by the American Craft Museum in New York in December 1988 and sponsored by Nestlé Chocolate. William Dufty's *Sugar Blues* was published in paperback by Warner Books in 1976. Marshall Efron lampoons Froot Loops in the film "A Chemical Feast," distributed by Benchmark Films, Inc. The Sugar Association's campaign was reported in "Taking the Guilt Out of Sweets," *The New York Times*, February 12, 1989. The Center for Science in the Public Interest publishes a useful poster, "How Sweet Is It? CSPI's Sugar Scoreboard," $3.95 (bulk rates available) from CSPI, 1501 16th Street, N.W., Washington, D.C. 20036, (202)332-9110. Objections to artificial sweeteners were reported in *The Wall Street Journal* ("New Sweeteners Head for the Sugar Bowl," by Alix M. Freedman, February 2, 1989), *Longevity* ("Sweet Fears," by Mary Lee Chin, June 1989), and *The New York Times* ("For Dieters With a Sweet Tooth, Scientists Offer New Choices," by Warren E. Leary, September 5, 1989). One of several studies documenting that many people have trouble absorbing fructose was done by C. M. F. Kneepkens et al., "Incomplete Intestinal Absorption of Fructose," *Archives of Diseases in Children* 59:735–38, August 1984. Sorbitol's link to abdominal pain was established by several studies, including N. K. Jain et al., "Sorbitol Intolerance in Adults," *American Journal of Gastroenterology* 1985; 80:678–81. The increase in Americans' consumption of high-fructose corn syrup was reported in *Self* in "Sweet Surrender," by Carl Lowe, December 1988. Anthony Cerami, Helen Vlassara, and Michael Brownlee describe how excess glucose may accelerate aging in "Glucose and Aging," *Scientific American*, vol. 225, no. 5, May 1987. Dr. C. Orian Truss pioneered treatment for chronic candidiasis and describes its role in digestive disorders in *The Missing Diagnosis* ($8.95 paperback plus shipping from The Missing Diagnosis, Inc., P.O. Box 26508, Birmingham, Alabama 35226). Another pioneer is Dr. William Crook, author of *The Yeast Connection* (New York: Vintage, 1987). Truss and Crook's theories are dismissed by *The Harvard Medical School Health Letter*, vol. 12, no. 4, February 1987. Modern methods of producing well-marbled meat are documented in Orville Schell's *Modern Meat* (New York: Random House, 1984). A *New York Times* editorial, "Secret Fat," February 21, 1989, cited a Center for Science in the Public Interest report on misleading labeling of supermarket meat. Studies linking a high-fat, low-fiber diet and various forms of gastrointestinal cancer are reviewed by M. Pariza in "Dietary Fat and Cancer Risk: Evidence and Research Needs," *Annual Review of Nutrition* 1988; 8:167–83. *The Paleolithic Prescription*, by S. Boyd Eaton, M.D., Marjorie Shostak, and Melvin Konner, M.D., Ph.D. (New York: Harper and Row, 1988), discusses findings that meat from free-ranging game animals has five times the proportion of polyunsaturated fat as supermarket meat. Eaton et al. cite studies such as "Fatty-Acid Ratios in Free-Living and Domestic Animals," by M. A. Crawford, *Lancet* I, 1968; 1329–33, and "Eating Quality of Meat Animal Products and Their Fat Content," by G. C. Smith and Z. L. Carpenter in the National Research Council's report, *Fat Content and Composition of Animal Products* (Washington, D.C.: National Academy of Sciences, 1976).

Fast Food

Marshall Efron critiques Potato Crisps and Kool-Aid in the film "A Chemical Feast," distributed by Benchmark Films, Inc. An ABC News special report entitled "America's Children: Diet of Danger," part of the "Burning Questions" series and broadcast December 29, 1988, documented the high fat, sugar, and salt content of junk food and fast food. In *The New England Journal of Medicine*, September 14, 1989, a report written by Connie Roberts for the nutrition committee of the Massachusetts Medical Society found that fast-food fish and chicken are loaded with vast amounts of hidden fat. *The Fast-Food Guide*, by Michael F. Jacobson, Ph.D., and Sarah Fritschner (New York: Workman Publishing, 1986) lists the ingredients of most popular fast foods.

Antacids

The important Swedish study documenting the near-uselessness of antacids for gastritis is "Absence of Therapeutic Benefit from Antacids or Cimetidine in Non-Ulcer Dyspepsia," by Olof Nyrén, M.D., et al.

---

in *The New England Journal of Medicine*, vol. 314, no. 6, February 6, 1986. The Public Citizen Health Research Group's study of over-the-counter medications is *Over the Counter Pills That Don't Work* (New York: Pantheon, 1983). Alfred Goodman Gilman, Louis S. Goodman, and Alfred Gilman describe the deleterious effects of antacids' ingredients in *The Pharmacological Basis of Therapeutics* (New York: Macmillan, 1980). Michael A. Weiner, Ph.D., connects Alzheimer's disease and aluminum in *Reducing the Risk of Alzheimer's* (Briarcliff Manor, New York: Stein & Day, 1987).

CHAPTER FOUR

A good general discussion of food allergy and intolerance appears in "Food Sensitivity," by A. Stewart Truswell, *British Medical Journal* 291:951–55, October 5, 1985. An unusual case in which gluten intolerance turned out to be the cause of lupus is documented by A. K. Rustgi and M. A. Peppercorn in "Gluten-Sensitive Enteropathy and Systemic Lupus Erythematosus," *Archives of Internal Medicine*, July 1988, vol. 148, no. 7, 1583–84. A definitive source on food allergy and intolerance is *Basics of Food Allergy*, by James C. Breneman, M.D. (Springfield, Illinois: Charles C. Thomas, 1984).

Lactose
A useful explanation of lactose intolerance appears in *Milk Intolerance Due to Lactase Deficiency*, by Gary M. Gray, M.D., a fact sheet available free of charge from National Digestive Diseases Education and Information Clearinghouse, Box NDDIC, Bethesda, Maryland 20892, (301)469-6344. Custy F. Fernandes and Khem M. Shahani's study of using lactobacilli to treat lactose intolerance, "Modulation of Lactose Intolerance with Lactobacilli and Other Microbial Supplements," was published in the *Journal of Applied Nutrition*, early in 1990. The information in the sidebar "Incidence of Lactose Intolerance in Adults" was drawn from "The Acceptability of Milk and Milk Products in Populations with a High Prevalence of Lactose Intolerance," a supplement to vol. 48, no. 4 of the *American Journal of Clinical Nutrition*, October 1988. The information in the sidebar "Which Foods Contain Lactose?" appeared in "Diet Therapy on Adult Lactose Malabsorption: Present Practices" by Jack D. Welsh, M.D., in the *American Journal*

of Clinical Nutrition, vol. 31, April 1978, 592–96. Reprinted by permission.

Fructose

One of several studies documenting that many people have trouble absorbing fructose was done by C. M. F. Kneepkens et al. in "Incomplete Intestinal Absorption of Fructose," *Archives of Diseases in Children* 59:735–38, August 1984. Jeffrey S. Hyams and A. Leichtner documented that apple juice can cause diarrhea and intestinal disorders in infants in "Apple Juice: An Unappreciated Cause of Chronic Diarrhea," *American Journal of Diseases of Children* 1985; 139:503–5. The National Center for Health Statistics' calculations are based on an analysis of the second National Health and Nutrition Examination Survey (NHANES II) by Blossom H. Patterson, M.A., and Gladys Block, Ph.D., published as "Food Choices and the Cancer Guidelines" in *American Journal of Public Health,* vol. 78, no. 3, March 1988.

Gluten

The history and symptoms of celiac sprue are described in "Coeliac [sic] Sprue: A Centennial Overview 1888–1988" by Michael N. Marsh and Duncan E. Loft, *Digestive Diseases* 1988; 6:216–28. Celiac sprue's ability to mimic other diseases is described by Fergus Shanahan, M.D., and Wilfred Weinstein, M.D., in "Extending the Scope in Celiac Disease," in *The New England Journal of Medicine,* September 22, 1988. The researchers in Pavia, Italy, who found that the Eucharist was problematic for children with celiac disease, described their research in a letter to *The New England Journal of Medicine,* which was reprinted in a collection of such letters entitled *Hunan Hand and Other Ailments,* edited and compiled by Shirley Blotnick Moskow (Boston: Little, Brown, 1987). Besides quinoa, another Aztec grain is amaranth, described by William Mueller in "Amaranth: Grain of the Gods," in *East/West* Magazine, June 1989.

Candida

Dr. C. Orian Truss pioneered treatment for chronic candidiasis and describes its role in digestive disorders in *The Missing Diagnosis* ($8.95 paperback plus shipping from The Missing Diagnosis, Inc., P.O. Box 26508, Birmingham, Alabama 35226). Another pioneer is Dr. William Crook, author of *The Yeast Connection* (New York: Vintage, 1987). The widespread use of antibiotics and growth hormones in raising farm

---

animals is documented in Orville Schell's *Modern Meat* (New York: Random House, 1984). "New Study Adds to Antibiotic Debate" (*Science* 226:818) describes a study conducted by Scott A. Holmberg et al. at the Centers for Disease Control that established a link between the use of antibiotics in cattle feed and human illness by tying 18 cases of diarrheal illness to antibiotic-resistant bacteria in beef.

CHAPTER FIVE

Water

F. Batmanghelidj, M.D., describes using water to treat over 3,000 prisoners in an Iranian jail with ulcer symptoms in "A New and Natural Method of Treatment of Peptic Ulcer Disease," *Journal of Clinical Gastroenterology*, May/June 1983; 5:203–5.

Fiber

Denis P. Burkitt and Hugh C. Trowell first described the link between a high-fiber diet and low incidence of bowel cancer in *Refined Carbohydrate Foods and Disease: Some Implications of Dietary Fibre* (London and New York: Academic Press, 1975). Trowell's findings are cited by Alan Silman and Jean Marr in their essay "A Better Western Diet: What Can Be Achieved?" in *Dietary Fibre, Fibre-Depleted Foods and Disease*, edited by Hugh C. Trowell, Denis Burkitt, and Kenneth Heaton (New York: Academic Press, 1985). A good general article on the various types of dietary fiber and their role in prevention of digestive disease is "Dietary Fiber," by Bernard Levin, M.D., and David Horwitz, M.D., *Medical Clinics of North America*, September 1979, vol. 63, no. 5, 1043–55. The advent of psyllium as a cereal was reported in *The New York Times* ("Flirting with Health Claim, Kellogg Announces a Cereal," August 31, 1989, and "Psyllium in Cereal: Unknown Territory," September 6, 1989) and *The Wall Street Journal* ("Cereal Makers Using Psyllium Face Scrutiny by FDA," September 1, 1989). The case of the 75-year-old man with a bran bezoar was reported in a letter from Stanley G. Cooper, M.D., and Edward J. Tracey, M.D., to *The New England Journal of Medicine* 32; 17:1148–49, April 27, 1989. The information in the sidebar "How to Eat More Fiber" originally appeared in *Nutrition Action Healthletter*, the newsletter of the Center for Science in the Public Interest, and is reprinted by permission in an updated form.

Calcium

Dr. Cedric Garland and Dr. Frank Garland describe the roles of calcium and fiber in preventing colon cancer in *The Calcium Connection*, which they wrote with Ellen Thro (New York: Simon and Schuster, 1989). Alexander Walker also discusses calcium and fiber in his essay "Mineral Metabolism" in *Dietary Fibre, Fibre-Depleted Foods and Disease*, edited by Hugh C. Trowell, Denis Burkitt, and Kenneth Heaton (New York: Academic Press, 1985). Research on dissolution rates of commercially available calcium tablets was conducted between March 1987 and January 1988 by Dr. Ralph Shangraw, chairman of the department of pharmaceutics at the University of Maryland School of Pharmacy, and reported in *The New York Times*, January 27, 1988.

Vegetables and Herbs

In "The Well-Traveled Tomato" (*Natural History*, June 1989), Raymond Sokolov cites M. A. Stevens, whose University of California, Davis, study analyzed the tomato's nutritional value. A good general article on the nutritional value of sea vegetables is "The Noble Sea Vegetables: Algae with Image Problems," by Gail Forman, *The New York Times*, August 31, 1988. The collaborative study by the National Cancer Institute and Chinese scientists is "Allium Vegetables and Reduced Risk of Stomach Cancer," by Wei-Cheng You, William J. Blot, et al., *Journal of the National Cancer Institute*, vol. 81, no. 2, January 18, 1989. The digestive benefits of bitter herbs are detailed in *The Scientific Validation of Herbal Medicine*, by Daniel B. Mowrey, Ph.D. (Lehi, Utah: Cormorant Books, 1986), and in *Herbal Medicine*, by Rudolf Fritz Weiss, M.D. (Beaconsfield, England: Beaconsfield Publishers, Ltd., distributed in the United States by Medicina Biologia, 4830 N.E. 32nd Avenue, Portland, Oregon 97211). A good general article on bitter herbs is "A Matter of Taste," by Mark Blumenthal, *East/West*, April 1989.

Fermented Foods

The differences in lactobacillus content of commercial brands of yogurt were confirmed by D. H. Wytock and J. A. Di Palma's study, *American Journal of Clinical Nutrition* 47; 3:454–57, March 1988. Ann Marie Cunningham gave me the recipe for homemade yogurt, which she has used for years. The recipe for lassi is adapted from Julie Sahni's *Classic Indian Cooking* (New York: William Morrow, 1980).

CHAPTER SIX

The following organizations can help you locate a nutritionally-oriented medical doctor who takes a preventive approach:

American Academy of Environmental Medicine
P.O.Box 16106
Boulder, Colorado 80216
(303)622-9755

American College for Advancement in Medicine
23121 Verdugo Drive, Suite 204
Laguna Hills, California 92653
(714)583-7666

American Holistic Medical Association
2727 Fairview Avenue East, #D
Seattle, Washington 98102
(206)322-6842

Foundation for the Advancement of Innovative Medicine
P.O. Box 338
Kinderhook, New York 12106-0338
(800)462-FAIM

Thorough discussions of malabsorption are found in "When All That's Eaten Isn't Absorbed," by Jerry S. Trier, M.D. (*Emergency Medicine*, January 15, 1987), and "Workup of the Patient with Malabsorption," by Ingram M. Roberts, M.D. (*Postgraduate Medicine* 81; 7:32–42, May 15, 1987). The review by C. C. Tennant, M.D., of the "Psychosocial Causes of Duodenal Ulcer" appeared in the *Australian and New Zealand Journal of Psychiatry* 1988; 22:195–201. The number of chickens contaminated with *Salmonella* was reported in *Science News* (June 3, 1989), in a report on John R. DeLoach and his colleagues at the U.S. Department of Agriculture, who sweetened the drinking water of broiler chickens with lactose, dramatically increasing their ability to resist *Salmonella* infection.

Sushi
The case of the 24-year-old man who was infected with nematodes after eating homemade sushi was reported by Murray Wittner, M.D.,

Ph.D., et al. in "Eustrongylidiasis—A Parasitic Infection Acquired by Eating Sushi" in *The New England Journal of Medicine*, vol. 320, no. 17:1124–26, April 27, 1989. Several doctors' responses to this case and to the risks posed by sushi appear in the *Journal*'s issue for September 28, 1989, vol. 321, no. 13:900–901. The Centers for Disease Control's recommendation that adequate freezing will kill parasites in raw fish appears in a letter to the *Journal* from Peter M. Schwantz, V.M.D., Ph.D. ("The Dangers of Eating Raw Fish," in vol. 320, no. 17:1143–45, April 27, 1989).

Giardiasis

Sales of purification equipment and services were reported in "Concern Over Water Safety Is Growing," by Michael deCourcy Hinds, *The New York Times*, March 25, 1989. The National Wildlife Federation (1400 16th Street, N.W., Washington, D.C. 20036-2266, (292)637-3750) published its study of water-supply pollution, *Danger on Tap*, by Norman L. Dean, in October 1988. The information on giardiasis is based on "Teaching Rounds: Giardiasis," *Hospital Medicine*, August 1988; "Giardiasis," by Neal R. Holtan, M.D., M.P.H., *Postgraduate Medicine* 83; 5:54–61, April 1988; and Jane E. Brody's "Personal Health" column, *The New York Times*, October 27, 1988. Dr. Leo Galland reported to the 1989 meeting of the American College of Gastroenterology that in his study of 197 patients thought to have irritable bowel syndrome, 48 percent actually had giardiasis. According to *The New York Times* ("Test Unmasks a Parasitic Disease," by Jane E. Brody, October 26, 1989), Dr. Galland estimates that about 24 percent of IBS patients nationwide probably have giardiasis. The number of travelers to Third World countries who are afflicted with traveler's diarrhea was reported in Jane E. Brody's "Personal Health" column, *The New York Times*, June 15, 1989. The case of a 14-month-old who contracted a parasitic infection from aquarium water occurred in Missouri and was reported in the Centers for Disease Control's *Morbidity and Mortality Weekly Report*, September 15, 1989; 38:617–19.

Gender

New findings that demonstrate the role of gastric hormones during pregnancy are described by Kerstin Uvnäs-Moberg, M.D., Ph.D., in "The Gastrointestinal Tract in Growth and Reproduction," *Scientific American*, July 1989. The effect of endometriosis on digestion is described in *Overcoming Endometriosis*, by Mary Lou Ballweg and the Endometriosis Association (New York: Congdon & Weed, 1987).

Surgery

Kuoung-Yi Liaw et al. describe the aftereffects of intestinal surgery in "The Nutritional Consequences of Gastric and Pancreatic Surgery," *Journal of the Formosan Medical Association* 1984; 83; 11:1105–12. L. M. De Lucia and R. P. Calabria present a critique of gastroplasty in "Gastroplasty for Obesity. A Critical Analysis of Techniques, Complications, and Results," *Clinical Nutrition* 1986, supplement to vol. 5, 67–72. Harvey N. Mandell, M.D., presents another critique in *Postgraduate Medicine* 82; 1:28–32, July 1987. A case of night blindness after intestinal surgery was reported in "Night Vision Impaired After Jejunoileal Bypass Surgery," *Internal Medicine News* 19; 4:77. The deleterious effects of comfrey tea on the liver are described by Nancy Bach, M.D., et al. in "Comfrey Herb Tea–Induced Hepatic Veno-Occlusive Disease," *American Journal of Medicine* 87:97–99, July 1989. The case of the doctor who overdosed on fiber was reported by Fred Saibil, M.D., in a letter to *The New England Journal of Medicine* 320; 9:599, March 2, 1989. A good primer on Chinese medicine is *The Web That Has No Weaver*, by Ted J. Kaptchuk, O.M.D. (New York: Congdon & Weed, 1983).

Stool Analysis

Vaughn M. Bryant, Jr., professor of anthropology and biology at Texas A & M University, specializes in chemical and content analyses of coprolites, or fossilized feces. He describes the process of soaking coprolites in "The Role of Coprolite Analysis in Archeology," *Bulletin of the Texas Archeological Society*, vol. 45, 1974, and in "The Coprolites of Man," *Scientific American*, vol. 232, no. 1, January 1975. Hugh C. Trowell's ideas concerning colon cancer appear in *Western Diseases: Their Emergence and Prevention*, edited by Hugh C. Trowell and Denis P. Burkitt (Cambridge, Massachusetts: Harvard University Press, 1981). The phenomenon of black stools resulting from Hydrox cookies and other foods is cited in a letter from Stephen Sulkes, M.D., to *The New England Journal of Medicine*, reprinted in *Hunan Hand and Other Ailments*, edited and compiled by Shirley Blotnick Moskow (Boston: Little, Brown, 1987). A good general discussion of the CDSA appears in "Comprehensive Digestive Stool Analysis," by Stephen A. Barrie, N.D., in *A Textbook of Natural Medicine*, edited by S. Barrie, J. Piz-

---

zorno, and M. Murray (Seattle: JBC Press, 1986). R. M. Jaffe, M.D., Ph.D., et al. discuss some of the ways that the Hemoccult test can be confounded in "False-Negative Stool Occult Blood Tests Caused by Ingestion of Ascorbic Acid (Vitamin C)," *Annals of Internal Medicine* 1975; 83:824–26. J. M. Jaffe and W. Zierdt discuss new testing methods in "A New Occult Blood Test Not Subject to False-Negative Results From Reducing Substances," *The Journal of Laboratory and Clinical Medicine* 93; 5:879–86, May 1979. More information on the Heidelberg test is available from Heidelberg International Division, Electro-Medical Devices, Inc., 6669 Peachtree Industrial Boulevard, Norcross, Georgia 30092. The Enterotest for diagnosing giardiasis is described in "Giardiasis," by Neal R. Holtan, M.D., M.P.H., *Postgraduate Medicine* 83; 5:54–61, April 1988.

CHAPTER SEVEN

Food Fallacies and Fasting
One study demonstrating that starch blockers do not result in weight loss is "Starch Blockers—Their Effect on Calorie Absorption From a High-Starch Meal," by G. W. bo-Linn et al., *New England Journal of Medicine* 307:1413–16, December 2, 1982. The "Fit for Life" diet is described in *Fit for Life*, by Harvey Diamond and Marilyn Diamond (New York: Warner Books, 1985). The father of food combining, Herbert M. Shelton, explained his ideas in *Food Combining Made Easy* (San Antonio, Texas: Willow Publishing, 1982). A critique of Shelton and the Diamonds, entitled *"Fit for Life:* Some Notes on the Book and Its Roots" by James J. Kenney, Ph.D., R.D., appears in *Nutrition Forum* 3; 8:57–59, August 1986. Professor Arnold Ehret explained his ideas in *Rational Fasting* (Beaumont, California; Ehret Literature Publishing Company, 1965). Rudolph Ballantine, M.D., explains the daily fast in his book, *Diet and Nutrition* (Honesdale, Pennsylvania: The Himalayan International Institute, 1978), pages 383–85.

Food Supplements and Vegetarianism
Statistics on annual sales of vitamins and nutritional supplements come from the Council for Responsible Nutrition, 2100 M Street N.W., Suite 602, Washington, D.C. 20037-1207, (202)872-1488. The cancer risk associated with high body levels of iron was documented by

R. Stevens et al. in "Body Iron and the Risk of Cancer," *The New England Journal of Medicine* 1988; 319:1047–52. The American Dietetic Association's opinion appears on the Vegetarian Resource Group's poster, "Vegetarianism in a Nutshell." According to *The Lancet,* March 22, 1986, page 695, a survey of vegetarians conducted by J. W. T. Dickerson of the University of Surrey and Dr. G. J. Davies of South Bank Polytechnic found that constipation, appendicitis, irritable bowel syndrome, gallstones, angina pectoris, hemorrhoids, varicose veins, and iron-deficiency anemia were all "more common among omnivores and where these conditions did appear in vegetarians they occurred later in life." One study noting that vegetarianism might reduce risk of cancer is "Increased Green and Yellow Vegetable Intake and Lowered Cancer Deaths in an Elderly Population," by G. Colditz et al., *American Journal of Clinical Nutrition* 1985; 4:32–36.

Stress

In *An Invisible Spectator* (New York: Weidenfeld & Nicolson, 1989), a biography of the writer Paul Bowles, author Christopher Sawyer-Laucanno describes Bowles's upbringing according to Fletcher's principles. The dental-school study of the digestive benefits of careful chewing is "Oral Digestion of a Complex-Carbohydrate Cereal: Effects of Stress and Relaxation on Physiological and Salivary Measures," by Donald R. Morse et al., *American Journal of Clinical Nutrition* 1989; 49:97–105. A good general discussion of stress and its effect on digestion is "Understanding Stress" in *Living Healthy* (vol. 6, no. 1, January 1985), a publication of the American Digestive Disease Society (7720 Wisconsin Avenue, Bethesda, Maryland 20814). This article includes the Social Readjustment Rating Scale, a list of 43 life events that cause stress. Another good general source is *Stress and Nutrition,* by Judith Swarth, M.S., R.D., a booklet in the Health Media of America Nutrition Series (Health Media of America, Inc., 11300 Sorrento Valley Road, Suite 250, San Diego, California 92121). The percentage of gastrointestinal disorders in which stress plays a part is cited by H. Richard Waranch, Ph.D., in "Relaxation Therapy," *Current Management of Inflammatory Bowel Diseases,* edited by Theodore M. Bayless (Toronto: Decker, 1989). Dr. Herbert Benson's book *The Relaxation Response* was published by William Morrow in New York in 1975. The Texas A & M University study that found that eliminating caffeine and sugar cuts down on stress is "Impact of a Dietary Change on Emotional

Distress," by L. Christiansen et al., *Journal of Abnormal Psychology* 1985; 94:565–79. Dr. Mark Schwartz presents his analogy in *Biofeedback: A Practitioner's Guide*, by Mark S. Schwartz et al. (New York: Academic Press, 1985).

Exercise

The sources for the numbers of Americans who exercise are the National Sporting Goods Association and Bicycle Market Research Institute. The largest study ever carried out linking exercise and longevity was led by Dr. Steven N. Blair at the Institute for Aerobics Research and the Cooper Clinic in Dallas, Texas, and reported in *The New York Times* ("Exercise and Longevity: A Little Goes a Long Way," by Philip J. Hilts, November 3, 1989). The study by Donald O. Castell et al. which found that running can cause heartburn was "Gastroesophageal Reflux Induced by Exercise in Healthy Volunteers," published in the June 23–30, 1989, issue of the *Journal of the American Medical Association* (vol. 261; 24:3599–3601), and reported in *The New York Times* ("Study Says Running Can Cause Heartburn," July 6, 1989). Glaxo's promotion of Zantac to prevent heartburn in runners was reported in William Stockton's "Fitness" column in *The New York Times* ("Heartburn for Fun and Profit: A Saga," May 22, 1989). Two useful books that explain and show in photographs how to do yoga exercises that aid digestion are Richard Hittleman's *Yoga: 28-Day Exercise Plan* (New York: Workman Publishing Company, 1969), and *Yoga for a New Age,* by Bob Smith and Linda Boudreau Smith (Smith Productions, 2116 North 122 Street, Seattle, Washington 98133).

Meditation

The Western Buddhist Order's method of meditation was reported in the *Manchester Guardian Weekly,* January 29, 1989. For more information on meditation techniques, see *How to Meditate,* by Lawrence LeShan (Boston: Little, Brown, 1974), and *Healing from Within,* by Dennis T. Jaffe, Ph.D. (New York: Simon and Schuster, 1980).

Chiropractic

The investigations linking spinal abnormalities to digestive disorders were conducted by Henry Winsor, M.D., and are known as "the Winsor autopsies." Dr. Winsor described his findings in "Sympathetic Segmental Disturbances 11: The Evidence of the Association in Dissected Cadavers, of Visceral Disease with Vertebrae Deformities of the

Same Sympathetic Segments," *Medical Times*, 49:1–7, November 1921. Excellent explanations of the basic principles of chiropractic and homeopathic care are found in *Alternatives in Healing*, by Simon Mills, M.A., and Steven J. Finando, Ph.D. (New York: New American Library, 1988).

Homeopathy

Homeopathy: Medicine for the 21st Century, by Dana Ullman (Berkeley, California: North Atlantic Books, 1988), and "Homeopathy: A Special Report," by Richard Leviton (*Yoga Journal*, March/April 1989), cover the history, principles, and current issues in homeopathy. Jacques Benveniste et al. published their original study, "Human Basophil Degranulation Triggered by Very Dilute Antiserum Against IgE" in *Nature* 333:816–18, June 30, 1988. The editors' caveat appears on page 787 of the same issue. The report of the team of investigators, along with Benveniste's reply, appeared in *Nature* 334:287–91, July 28, 1989. For more information about homeopathy, contact the Foundation for Homeopathic Education and Research, 5916 Chabot Cross, Oakland, California 94618, (415)420-8791.

Biofeedback

A basic overview of biofeedback and biofeedback training appears in "Biofeedback and States of Consciousness" by Elmer E. Green and Alyce M. Green, in *Handbook of States of Consciousness*, edited by Benjamin B. Wolman and Montague Ullman (New York: Van Nostrand Reinhold, 1986). The study commissioned by the U.S. Army is *Enhancing Human Performance*, edited by Daniel Druckman and John A. Swets (Washington, D.C.: National Academy Press, 1988). Among the studies showing biofeedback's positive effect on gastrointestinal disorders are "Management of Anal Incontinence by Biofeedback," by James MacLeod, *Gastroenterology* 1987; 93:291–94; "Biofeedback and Behavioral Approaches to Disorders of the Gastrointestinal Tract," by Paul R. Latimer, *Psychotherapy and Psychosomatics* 1981; 36; 3-4:200–212; "Behavioral Medicine Approaches to Gastrointestinal Disorders," by William E. Whitehead and Linda S. Bosmajian, *Journal of Consulting and Clinical Psychology* 50; 6:972–83, December 1982; "Biofeedback Treatment for Headaches, Raynaud's Disease, Essential Hypertension, and Irritable Bowel Syndrome: A Review of the Long-Term Follow-Up Literature," by Martin R. Ford, *Biofeedback and Self-Regulation* 7; 4:521–36, December 1982. Dr. Steven L. Fahrion, director of the Voluntary Controls Program at the Menninger Foundation, warns that "research on biofeedback, while generally positive, is often not as positive as the results obtained by competent clinicians. In fact, it often lags two to five years behind the best clinical work."

Hypnotherapy

A Primer of Clinical Hypnosis, by Barbara DeBetz, M.D., and Gérard Sunnen, M.D. (Littleton, Massachusetts: PSG Publishing Company, 1985) describes medical use of hypnosis. Two new studies document hypnotherapy's effectiveness in treating gastrointestinal disorders: "Hypnotherapy in Severe Irritable Bowel Syndrome: Further Experience," by P. J. Whorwell et al., *Gut* 1987; 28:423–25, and "Controlled Trial of Hypnotherapy in Relapse Prevention of Duodenal Ulceration," by S. M. Colgan, E. B. Faragher, and P. J. Whorwell, *The Lancet*, June 11, 1988. In the June 1989 issue of *The American Journal of Psychiatry*, David Spiegel, M.D., a psychiatrist at Stanford Medical School, describes his research indicating that hypnosis can suppress the brain's perception of pain. His work is summarized in *The New York Times* ("Study Finds Hypnosis Can Suppress Brain's Perception of Pain," by Daniel Goleman, June 22, 1989). The study showing the effectiveness of self-help books was published in the June 1989 issue of *The Journal of Consulting and Clinical Psychology*, and reported in *The New York Times* ("Feeling Gloomy? A Good Self-Help Book May Actually Help," July 6, 1989).

CHAPTER EIGHT

Intestinal Gas

François Rabelais's Queen appears in *The Histories of Gargantua and Pantagruel* (London: Penguin Books, 1955). Geoffrey Chaucer first used the word "fart" in "The Miller's Tale," one of *The Canterbury Tales* (*The Portable Chaucer*, London: Penguin Books, 1949). A basic description of intestinal gas and digestive problems associated with it appears in *Gas in the Digestive Tract*, by Harris R. Clearfield, M.D., NIH Publication No. 85-883, a fact sheet available free of charge from National Digestive Diseases Education and Information Clearinghouse, Box NDDIC, Bethesda, Maryland 20892, (301)469-6344. Another excellent overview is "Intestinal Gas: Insights into an Ancient

Malady," by Naresh K. Jain, M.D., James S. Vela, M.D., and C. S. Pitchumoni, M.D. For more information about *Candida* infections, consult Dr. C. Orian Truss's *The Missing Diagnosis* ($8.95 paperback plus shipping from The Missing Diagnosis, Inc., P.O. Box 26508, Birmingham, Alabama 35226), or Dr. William Crook's *The Yeast Connection* (New York: Vintage, 1987). Studies of the gas-forming potential of various foods for astronauts were carried out by Dr. Judith McBride at the U.S. Department of Agriculture. The fact that simethicone is ineffective in the lower gastrointestinal tract, whereas activated charcoal does seem to relieve intestinal gas and abdominal discomfort, is documented by N. K. Jain, M.D., et al. in *Annals of Internal Medicine* 105:61–62, July 1986. Herbs that reduce intestinal gas are mentioned in *Herbal Medicine*, by Rudolf Fritz Weiss, M.D. (Beaconsfield, England: Beaconsfield Publishers, Ltd., distributed in the United States by Medicina Biologia, 4830 N.E. 32nd Avenue, Portland, Oregon 97211), and in *The Scientific Validation of Herbal Medicine*, by Daniel B. Mowrey, Ph.D. (Lehi, Utah: Cormorant Books, 1986).

Hiccups

Anecdotal evidence of the effectiveness of household remedies for hiccups, including granulated sugar and vinegar, is cited by Edgar G. Engleman, M.D., of the University of California School of Medicine, James Lankton, M.D., and Barbara Lankton, M.D., of the University of Miami School of Medicine, Aurelia D. Schisel and Roy S. Rhodes, M.S., of the University of Southern California School of Medicine, George Margolis, M.D., of Dartmouth Medical School, Jay Howard Herman, M.D., and David S. Nolan in letters to *The New England Journal of Medicine*. These letters were reprinted in a collection entitled *Hunan Hand and Other Ailments*, edited and compiled by Shirley Blotnick Moskow (Boston: Little, Brown, 1987). W. O. Jones et al. of the New York University School of Medicine have reported that biotin may relieve intractable hiccups.

Heartburn

Statistics on the frequency of heartburn appear in *Heartburn Across America*, a Gallup poll sponsored by Glaxo, Inc. A comprehensive fact sheet entitled *Heartburn*, by Donald O. Castell, M.D. (NIH Publication No. 86-882), is available free of charge from National Digestive Diseases Education and Information Clearinghouse, Box NDDIC, Bethesda, Maryland 20892, (301)469-6344. The study by Donald O. Castell et al. which found that running can cause heartburn was "Gastroesophageal Reflux Induced by Exercise in Healthy Volunteers," published in the June 23–30, 1989, issue of the *Journal of the American Medical Association,* vol. 261; 24:3599–3601. A summary of and comment on a recent Dutch study showing the effectiveness of bismuth in treating heartburn appeared in *Gastroenterology* 95; 4:1145–46. The usefulness of acid-suppressants is described by Daniel W. Murphy, M.D., and Donald O. Castell, M.D., in "Pathogenesis and Treatment of Gastroesophageal Reflux Disease," *Medical Times,* November 1987.

Constipation

Figures on the incidence of constipation and money spent on laxatives appear in *Age Page: Constipation,* a fact sheet available free of charge from National Digestive Diseases Education and Information Clearinghouse, Box NDDIC, Bethesda, Maryland 20892, (301)469-6344. The number of doctors' prescriptions for laxatives was reported by G. Zaloga et al. in "Anaphylaxis Following Psyllium Ingestion," *Journal of Allergy and Clinical Immunology* 1984; 74:79–80. A summary of the causes of constipation appears in *What Is Constipation?,* by Marvin Schuster, M.D., another free fact sheet from the Clearinghouse. Alison Stephen's chapter on constipation in *Dietary Fibre, Fibre-Depleted Foods and Disease,* edited by Hugh C. Trowell, Denis Burkitt, and Kenneth Heaton (London: Academic Press, 1985), describes the connection between the Western diet and frequency of constipation. A handbook of colonics is *Colon Health: The Key to a Vibrant Life,* by Norman W. Walker, D.Sc., Ph.D. (published in 1979 by O'Sullivan Woodside & Company, 2218 East Magnolia, Phoenix, Arizona 85034). A long interview with V. E. Irons appeared in *The Healthview Newsletter,* 1:10; 1977. The outbreak of amebiasis in Colorado due to colonics is documented by Gregory R. Istre, M.D., et al. in "An Outbreak of Amebiasis Spread by Colonic Irrigation at a Chiropractic Clinic," *New England Journal of Medicine* 1982; 307:339–42. Other documentation of hazards associated with colonics is listed in *Alternative Therapies, Unproven Methods, and Health Fraud,* a selected annotated bibliography edited by Michaela Sullivan-Fowler, Terry Austin, and Arthur W. Hafner, Ph.D. (Chicago: American Medical Association, 1988).

Hemorrhoids

General discussion appears in *Hemorrhoids* by Jim Fordham, M.A. (NIH Publication No. 89-3021), a free fact sheet from National Digestive Diseases Education and Information Clearinghouse, Box NDDIC, Bethesda, Maryland 20892, (301)469-6344, and in "Hemorrhoids: Current Approaches to an Ancient Problem," by Edmund Leff, M.D., in *Postgraduate Medicine* 82: 7; November 15, 1987. A review of causes and conventional therapy appears in "Pruritus ani," by Edsel J. Aucoin, M.D. (*Postgraduate Medicine* 82:7; November 15, 1987). Gary Hitzig, M.D., of New York's Laser Medical Center, provided background on laser surgery. In *The People's Pharmacy* (New York: Avon, 1980), Joe Graedon describes the ingredients in and ineffectiveness of Preparation H and other popular hemorrhoid remedies. In *Hemorrhoids: A Cure and Preventive* (New York: William Morrow, 1980), Robert Lawrence Holt describes the link between the Western diet and incidence of hemorrhoids.

Irritable Bowel Syndrome

Figures on the incidence of IBS appear in "Psychological Management of IBS," by Thomas N. Wise, M.D., *Practical Gastroenterology* 10:3; May/June 1986. This article reflects the conventional view of IBS as psychosomatic in nature. More recent thinking is reported in "New Evidence Cites Overactive Nerves for Irritable Bowel," by Gina Kolata, *The New York Times*, February 2, 1988, and in *Relief from IBS*, by Elaine Fantle Shimberg (New York: M. Evans & Co., 1988). In a review published in *Gastroenterology*, July 1988, 232–41, Kenneth B. Klein of the University of North Carolina Medical School concludes that there is not enough evidence to support the effectiveness of any single drug for IBS. In "The Role of Fiber and Other Dietary Factors in IBS," *Practical Gastroenterology* 10; 2:51–56, March/April 1986, Gerald Friedman, M.D., reviews studies that have found that adding fiber to the diet relieves IBS. Dr. Leo Galland reported to the 1989 meeting of the American College of Gastroenterology that by using the mucus swab test, he found that of 197 patients thought to have irritable bowel syndrome, 48 percent actually had giardiasis. According to *The New York Times* ("Test Unmasks a Parasitic Disease," by Jane E. Brody, October 26, 1989), Dr. Galland estimates that about 24 percent of IBS patients nationwide probably have giardiasis. The quote from V. Alun Jones et al. appears in *Food and the Gut*, edited by J. O.

Hunter and V. Alun Jones (Philadelphia: Baillière Tindal, 1985). De Lamar Gibbons's diet is available from Dr. Gibbons at 204 Oregon Street, Kellogg, Idaho 83837. The Welsh study of peppermint oil's effectiveness is "Peppermint Oil for the Irritable Bowel Syndrome: A Multicentre Trial," by M. J. Dew, B. K. Evans, and J. Rhodes, *The British Journal of Clinical Practice* 38; 11–12: 394–98, November/December 1984. The study showing the effectiveness of hypnosis in treating IBS is "Hypnotherapy in Severe Irritable Bowel Syndrome: Further Experience," by P. J. Whorwell et al., *Gut* 1987; 28:423–25.

Herbal Medicine

The Indian Council of Medical Research's investigations of Ayurvedic remedies are described in "Pulse Reading, Herbs and Oil Massage," by Doug M. Podolsky and Cathy Sears, *American Health*, July/August 1988. In *The Food Pharmacy* (New York: Bantam, 1988), Jean Carper describes studies documenting garlic's medicinal properties. Another good source on herbal medicine is *The New Honest Herbal*, by Varro E. Tyler, M.D. (Philadelphia: George F. Stickley, 1988).

Acupuncture

Michio Kushi describes Chinese methods of diagnosis in *How to See Your Health: Book of Oriental Diagnosis* (New York: Japan Publications, Inc., 1980). Chinese medicine's definition of six different kinds of ulcers is cited in *The Web That Has No Weaver*, by Ted J. Kaptchuk (New York: Congdon & Weed, 1983). *Alternatives in Healing*, by Simon Mills, M.A., and Steven J. Finando, Ph.D. (New York: New American Library, 1988), includes an excellent description of the principles of acupuncture. *Scientific Bases of Acupuncture*, edited by Bruce Pomeranz and Gabriel Stux (New York: Springer-Verlag, 1988), summarizes Western, Chinese, and Japanese research documenting the mechanisms of acupuncture. Dr. Bruce Pomeranz was interviewed on "East Meets West," a documentary produced by Anne Lieberman for "Innovation," the public television science series. Dr. Gabriel Stux described his work in "Acupuncture in Gastroscopy," a paper presented at the World Congress of Acupuncture in 1987.

CHAPTER NINE

Appendicitis

Alexander Walker and Denis Burkitt's chapter on appendicitis in *Dietary Fibre, Fibre-Depleted Foods and Disease*, edited by Hugh C. Trowell, Denis Burkitt, and Kenneth Heaton (London: Academic Press, 1985), links appendicitis to the Western diet. Dr. George Crile's opinion on treating appendicitis appears in *Dissent in Medicine: Nine Doctors Speak Out* (Chicago: Contemporary Books, 1985).

Diarrhea

The Centers for Disease Control figures on diarrhea appeared in "Infant Diarrhea Kills Hundreds Yearly in U.S.," by William K. Stevens, *The New York Times*, December 9, 1988. Two basic sources on diarrhea are *Diarrhea: Infectious and Other Causes*, by Sidney F. Phillips, M.D. (NIH Publication No. 86-2749, free of charge from National Digestive Diseases Education and Information Clearinghouse, Box NDDIC, Bethesda, Maryland 20892, (301)469-6344), and "Differential Diagnosis: Diarrhea," by Jordan B. Weiss, M.D., *Hospital Medicine*, October 1988, 136–51. A good summary of the digestive benefits that breast milk confers on infants appears in "Breast-Feeding: Second Thoughts," by John W. Gerrard, D.M., *Pediatrics* 54; 6:757–64, December 1974. Children's limited ability to absorb fructose is documented in "Incomplete Intestinal Absorption of Fructose," by C. Kneepkens, R. Vink, and J. Fernandes, *Archives of Diseases in Children* 1984; 59:735–38. Jeffrey S. Hyams, M.D., et al. documented children's difficulty absorbing sorbitol in *American Journal of Diseases of Children* 1985; 139:503. According to Dr. Theodore Nash of the National Institute of Allergy and Infectious Diseases, the Centers for Disease Control studies show that about ten percent of youngsters aged one to three in a typical day care center are infected with *Giardia*. When these centers have outbreaks, the infection rate in this age group can rise to 30 percent or more. Current over-the-counter remedies for diarrhea are summarized in "New Treatments Promise a More Powerful Attack on Diarrhea," by Philip E. Ross, *The New York Times*, March 30, 1989. An early study of the effectiveness of bentonite is "The Value of Bentonite for Diarrhea," by Frederic Damrau, M.D., *Medical Annals of the District of Columbia* 30; 6:326–28, June 1961. The Canadian study on whey is "The Immunoenhancing Property of Dietary Whey Protein Concentrate," by G. Bounous, P. Kongshavn, and P. Gold, *Clinical Investigative Medicine* 1988; 11:271–78. The Australian study is "Remission of Diarrhea due to Cryptosporidiosis in an Immunodeficient Child Treated With Hyperimmune Bovine Colostrum," by S. Tzipori, D. Roberton, and C. Chapman, *Australian Medical Journal* 293:1276–77, November 15, 1986. Studies of the effectiveness of ozone in treating diarrhea in AIDS patients were reported in the *Dallas Times Herald*, October 27, 1988. The effect of lactobacilli on diarrhea is described in "Control of Diarrhea by Lactobacilli," by Custy F. Fernandes, Ph.D., Khem M. Shahani, Ph.D., and M. A. Amer, Ph.D., *Journal of Applied Nutrition* 1988; 40; 1:32–43. The use of fecal implants to restore colonic balance is described in "Bacteriotherapy for Chronic Relapsing Clostridium Difficile Diarrhea in Six Patients," by M. Tvede and J. Rask-Madsen, *The Lancet*, 1156–60, May 27, 1989.

Ulcers

The incidence of ulcers is the most recent estimate available from the National Center for Health Statistics. Basic information about ulcers appears in *About Stomach Ulcers*, by Juan-R. Malagelada, M.D. (NIH Publication No. 87–676), free from the National Digestive Diseases Education and Information Clearinghouse, Box NDDIC, Bethesda, Maryland 20892, (301)469-6344. The fact that "no acid, no ulcer" is a false dictum is explained in "Duodenal Bulb Acidity and the Natural History of Duodenal Ulceration," by D. D. Kerrigan, et al., *The Lancet*, 61–63, July 8, 1989. The role of prostaglandins in preventing ulcers is explained in "Peptic Ulcer Disease, Cytoprotection, and Prostaglandins," an editorial by Steven C. Fiske, M.D., in the *Archives of Internal Medicine* 148:2112–13, October 1988, and "Prostaglandins in Peptic Ulcer Disease," by Donald E. Wilson, *Postgraduate Medicine* 81; 4:309–16, March 1987. Nicotine gum's role in exacerbating ulcers is documented in Karl Brandspigel, M.D., and Mark M. Walsh, M.D., in a letter to the *Archives of Internal Medicine* 147:1001, May 1987. An Australian study which found that up to 80 percent of gastric ulcers are caused by smoking and daily ingestion of analgesic and antiinflammatory drugs is "Environmental Factors in Aetiology of Chronic Gastric Ulcer: A Case Control Study of Exposure Variables Before the First Symptoms," by J. H. McIntosh, Karen Byth, and D. W. Piper, *Gut* 1985; 26:789–98. D. W. Piper et al. also conducted the study that found that marital separation or divorce may reactivate duodenal ulcers, reported in *Gut* 1987; 28:533–40. Milk's adverse effect on ulcers is documented by N. Kumar et al. in "Effect of Milk on Patients with Duodenal Ulcers," *British Medical Journal* 1986; 293:666. Dr. Barry J. Marshall describes his work in "Antimicrobial Therapy for Peptic Diseases: An Interview with Barry J. Marshall, M.D.," by Steve Stiles, *Internal Medicine* 8; 12:138–157, November 1987. H. Humphreys et al. found that bismuth eradicates *C. pylori*, *Gut* 1988; 29:279–83. Tea's effect on stomach acid production is described in "Effect of Tea on Gastric Acid Secretion," by P. Dubey et al., *Digest of Digestive Science* 29:202–206, March 1984. The study that infused pepper directly into ulcer patients' stomachs was "Spicy Food and the Stomach," by David Y. Graham et al., *Journal of the American Medical Association* 206; 23:3473–75, December 16, 1988. The Indian study using chili peppers was reported in the *British Journal of Medicine* 1984; 288:1804. The benefits of fiber are reported in "Prophylactic Effect of Dietary Fibre in Duodenal Ulcer Disease," by A. Rydning et al., *The Lancet*, 736–38, October 2, 1982. Jean Carper documents cabbage's healing powers in *The Food Pharmacy* (New York: Bantam, 1988). F. Batmanghelidj, M.D., describes using water to treat over 3,000 prisoners in an Iranian jail with ulcer symptoms in "A New and Natural Method of Treatment of Peptic Ulcer Disease," *Journal of Clinical Gastroenterology* 5:203–5, May/June 1983. R. Best et al. reported the beneficial effects of plantain bananas in the *British Journal of Pharmacology* 1984; 82:107–116. The benefits of zinc and vitamin A have been reported in "Effect of Zinc Sulfate on Experimental Human Gastric Ulcer," by N. Mann and P. Brawn, *Journal of the American College of Nutrition* 1988; 7:423, and in "Cytoprotective Effect of Vitamin A and Its Clinical Importance in the Treatment of Patients With Chronic Gastric Ulcer," by I. Patty et al., *International Journal of Tissue Reactions* 1983; 5:301–7. S. Szabo and C. Rogers discuss their findings on the benefits of fish oil in a letter to *The Lancet*, page 119, January 16, 1988. In "Endoscopic Controlled Trial of Four Drug Regimens in the Treatment of Chronic Duodenal Ulceration," Z. A. Kassir found that DGL healed ulcers faster than Tagamet or Zantac, *Irish Medical Journal* 1985; 78:153–56.

Inflammatory Bowel Disease

A basic description of IBD appears in *Inflammatory Bowel Disease,* by David B. Sachar, M.D., a free fact sheet from the National Digestive

Diseases Education and Information Clearinghouse, Box NDDIC, Bethesda, Maryland 20892, (301)469-6344. Kenneth Heaton's chapter on "Crohn's Disease and Ulcerative Colitis" in *Dietary Fibre, Fibre-Depleted Foods and Disease,* edited by Hugh C. Trowell, Denis Burkitt, and Kenneth Heaton (London: Academic Press, 1985), describes the link between IBD and the Western diet. Marvin Bush's activities were reported in "Bushes Enter a Glare, Warily but Unblinking," by Maureen Dowd, *The New York Times,* December 12, 1988. The possibility that IBD is caused by a virus or bacterium is discussed in an editorial, "Mycobacteria and Crohn's Disease," by S. J. Hampson, J. J. McFadden, and J. Hermon-Taylor in *Gut* 1988; 29:1017–19. Among the many studies that document the role of food intolerance in IBD is "Food Intolerance: A Major Factor in the Pathogenesis of Irritable Bowel Syndrome," by V. Alun Jones et al., *The Lancet* 1982; 2:1115–18. The study that found that Crohn's patients ate twice as much sugar is "Diet and Crohn's Disease: Characteristics of the Pre-Illness Diet," by J. R. Thornton, P. M. Emmett, and K. W. Heaton, *British Medical Journal* 1979; 279:762–64. In "Breakfast and Crohn's Disease," *British Medical Journal* 1977; 276:943–45, A. H. James found that Crohn's patients ate corn flakes more frequently. De Lamar Gibbons, M.D., has described his investigation of IBD in *The Care and Feeding of the Irritable Bowel,* available for $10.00 from Dr. Gibbons, 204 Oregon Street, Kellogg, Idaho 83837. The benefits of fiber are described by K. W. Heaton, J. R. Thornton, and P. M. Emmett in "Treatment of Crohn's Disease with an Unrefined-Carbohydrate, Fibre-Rich Diet," *British Medical Journal* 1979, vol. 2, no. 6193:764–66. The benefits of butyrates are described in "Treatment of Diversion Colitis with Short-Chain-Fatty Acid Irrigation," by James M. Harig, M.D., et al., *The New England Journal of Medicine* 320; 1:23–28, January 5, 1989.

Diverticular Disease

A good general description of diverticular disease appears in "New Hope for Those With Diverticular Disease," by Egon Weck, *FDA Consumer,* July/August 1987. Neil S. Painter and Denis P. Burkitt's article is "Diverticular Disease of the Colon: A Deficiency Disease of Western Civilization," *British Medical Journal* 1971; 2:450–54. Painter also has written on diverticular disease in his book, *Diverticular Disease of the Colon* (New Canaan, Connecticut: Keats Publishing, 1975), and in a chapter in *Dietary Fibre, Fibre-Depleted Foods and Disease,* edited by Hugh C. Trowell, Denis Burkitt, and Kenneth Heaton (New York: Academic Press, 1985). *Gut Reactions,* by W. Grant Thompson, M.D. (New York: Plenum, 1989), includes a comprehensive chapter on diverticular disease.

Gallbladder Disease

The incidence of gallstones and gallbladder surgery was reported in "Gasoline Additive Aids in Treating Gallstones," *The New York Times,* March 9, 1989. "Diet and Gallstone Formation" by Keith B. Taylor, M.D., summarizes recent research on the link between dietary habits and gallstones in *Nutrition and the M.D.,* vol. 12, no. 6, June 1986. The French study which reported that skipping meals is associated with a much higher incidence of gallstones appeared in the *British Medical Journal* 1981; 283:1435. F. Pixley et al., in "Effect of Vegetarianism on Development of Gallstones in Women," *British Medical Journal* 291:11–12, July 6, 1985, found that vegetarians had fewer gallstones. The San Antonio Heart Study and Dr. Andrew Diehl of the University of Texas Health Science Center report that taking steps to ward off heart disease also prevents gallstones. James C. Breneman, M.D., an expert on food intolerance, discusses its link with gallstones in *Basics of Food Allergy* (Springfield, Illinois: Charles C. Thomas, 1984). The Mayo Clinic's new treatment was reported in "Gasoline Additive Aids in Treating Gallstones," *The New York Times,* March 9, 1989. Martin Staritz et al. describe lithotripsy's use in Germany in a letter to *The Lancet,* July 18, 1987, page 155. Leslie J. Schoenfield, M.D., Ph.D., gives a longer description in "Treatment of Gallstones by Shock-Wave Lithotripsy," *Practical Gastroenterology* 11; 5:58–60, September/October 1987. The prairie dog study was conducted by Thomas H. Magnuson et al. at the Johns Hopkins University School of Medicine and reported in *Science News,* May 27, 1989. *The Harvard Medical School Health Letter* (11:4, February 1986) summarizes the known health benefits of fish oil. The study that found that moderate drinking protected men and women from gallstones was published in the *British Medical Journal* 1984; 288:1113. My patient who sought laser laparoscopic surgery consulted Eddie Joe Reddick, M.D., at the HCA Center for Research and Education, 220 25th Avenue North, Nashville, Tennessee 37203, (615)320-5050.

Cancer

The National Academy of Sciences, National Cancer Institute, and American Cancer Society all advocate a diet that is low in fat and high in fiber and vitamins A and C. A useful summary of studies of dietary factors in cancer appears in *Cancer and Nutrition,* by Elizabeth Somer, M.A., R.D., a booklet in the Health Media of America Nutrition Series (Health Media of America, Inc., 11300 Sorrento Valley Road, Suite 250, San Diego, California 92121). A more specific discussion of diet and colon cancer is found in *The Complete Book of Cancer Prevention,* by the editors of *Prevention* Magazine Health Books (Emmaus, Pennsylvania: Rodale Press, 1988). Many studies have documented the link between increasing incidence of lung, breast, colon, and prostate cancer in Japan and the Westernization of the Japanese diet. Two such studies are "A Case-Control Study of Prostatic Cancer with Reference to Dietary Habits," *Prostate* 1988; 12:179–190, and "Large Bowel Cancer in Hawaiian Japanese," by W. Haenszel et al., *Journal of the National Cancer Institute* 1973; 51:1765–99. The recent study on the benefits of fiber is "Effect of Wheat Fiber and Vitamins C and E on Rectal Polyps in Patients with Familial Adenomatous Polyposis," by Jerome J. DeCosse et al., *Journal of the National Cancer Institute* 81; 17:1290–97, September 6, 1989. This study was reported in "Stronger Data Show Fiber Reduces Colon Cancer," by Jane E. Brody, *The New York Times,* September 6, 1989. The largest study ever carried out linking exercise and longevity was led by Dr. Steven N. Blair at the Institute for Aerobics Research and the Cooper Clinic in Dallas, Texas, and reported in *The New York Times* ("Exercise and Longevity: A Little Goes a Long Way," by Philip J. Hilts, November 3, 1989). Dr. Cedric Garland and Dr. Frank Garland describe the roles of calcium and fiber in preventing colon cancer in *The Calcium Connection,* which they wrote with Ellen Thro (New York: Simon and Schuster, 1989). The recent study on the risks of ingesting too much iron is "Body Iron Stores and the Risk of Cancer," by Richard G. Stevens, Ph.D., et al., *The New England Journal of Medicine* 319; 16:1047–52, October 20, 1988. The study demonstrating the benefits of allium vegetables is "Allium Vegetables and Reduced Risk of Stomach Cancer," by Wei-Cheng You, William J. Blot, et al., *Journal of the National Cancer Institute,* vol. 81, no. 2, January 18, 1989. Linus Pauling and Ewan Cameron's original study of 100 patients with advanced cancer who were treated with vitamin C was published in *Proceedings of the Na-*

tional Academy of Science 1978; 75:4538. The Mayo Clinic's attempt to replicate this study appeared in *The New England Journal of Medicine* 1979; 301:687. Dr. Pauling criticized this study in a letter to the *Journal*, 1980; 302:694. Led by Charles G. Moertel, M.D., the Mayo Clinic conducted another study of 100 patients with advanced colorectal cancer, reported in *New England Journal of Medicine* 1985; 312:137. On September 5, 1989, Pauling lectured at the Mayo Clinic and declared that the second Mayo study also was flawed; *(Minneapolis Star-Tribune,* September 6, 1989). One of Dr. Khem Shahani's studies that found that lactobacilli inhibit tumor growth is "Antitumor Properties of Lactobacilli and Dairy Products Fermented by Lactobacilli," by B. A. Friend and K. M. Shahani, *Journal of Food Protection* 47; 9:717–23, September 1984. Michio Kushi explains the macrobiotic diet in *The Cancer Prevention Diet,* which he wrote with Alex Jack (New York: St. Martin's Press, 1983). Some critiques of the macrobiotic approach to cancer are listed in *Alternative Therapies, Unproven Methods, and Health Fraud,* a selected annotated bibliography edited by Michaela Sullivan-Fowler, Terry Austin, and Arthur W. Hafner, Ph.D. (Chicago: American Medical Association, 1988).

CHAPTER TEN

Food Poisoning

Three excellent overviews of the incidence of food poisoning, especially *Salmonella,* are in "Officials Call Microbes Most Urgent Food Threat," by William K. Stevens, *The New York Times,* March 28, 1989; "Salmonella," by Melanie Scheller, *Medical Selfcare,* July/August 1988; and "Foodborne Disease: A Needless Epidemic," by Beatrice Trum Hunter, *Clinical Ecology* 1987; 5; 1:23–31. The widespread use of antibiotics in animal feed is documented in Orville Schell's *Modern Meat* (New York: Random House, 1984). The epidemic of food poisoning due to contaminated shellfish was reported by Dale L. Morse, M.D., et al. in "Widespread Outbreaks of Clam- and Oyster-Associated Gastroenteritis," *The New England Journal of Medicine* 314; 11:678–81, March 13, 1986.

Travel

A comprehensive survey of the hazards of travel is "Travails of Travel," by Martin E. Gordon, M.D., in *Postgraduate Medicine*, vol. 84, no. 1, July 1988. Three overviews of the dangers of parasites are "Closing in on Protozoal Syndrome," *Emergency Medicine*, April 30, 1988; "Amebiasis," by Neal R. Holtan, M.D., M.P.H., *Postgraduate Medicine*, vol. 83, no. 8, June 1988; and "Giardiasis," also by Holtan, *Postgraduate Medicine*, vol. 83, no. 5, April 1988. The hazards of hot tap water are documented in "Heat Susceptibility of Bacterial Entero-pathogens," by Juan C. Bandres, M.D., et al., *Archives of Internal Medicine* 148:2261–63, October 1988. M. Koffler et al. reported Max von Pettenkofer's experiment in a letter to *The Lancet* ("Is Tannin Really Bactericidal?" August 26, 1989, page 503).

Children

Statistics on breast-feeding appeared in "The Importance of Mother's Milk," by Graham Carpenter (*Natural History*, August 1981) and in Jane E. Brody's "Personal Health" column in *The New York Times*, August 10, 1989. A summary of the nutritional advantages of breast milk is A. Stewart Truswell's "ABC of Nutrition: Infant Feeding," *British Medical Journal* 291:333–37, August 3, 1985. Another good overview is "Anti-infective Properties of Breast Milk," by J. K. Welsh, B.Sc., and J. T. May, Ph.D., *The Journal of Pediatrics* 94; 1:1–9, January 1979. The study which found that infants fed formula suffered six times more gastrointestinal illness than breast-fed babies is "Infant Formulas and Gastrointestinal Illness," by James S. Koopman et al., *American Journal of Public Health* 75:477–80, May 1985. The study that found that breast milk can kill parasites is "Human Milk Kills Parasitic Intestinal Protozoa," by Frances D. Gillin et al., *Science* 221:1290–92, September 23, 1983. Research on the effects of drinking alcohol on nursing infants was reported in "Caution About Alcohol For Nursing Mothers," *The New York Times*, August 17, 1989. The symptoms of infant protein intolerance are described by Stuart Berezi, M.D., et al. in *American Journal of Diseases of Children* 1989; 143:361. L. Lothe and T. Lindberg document the role of cow's milk protein in colic in "Cow's Milk Whey Protein Elicits Symptoms of Infantile Colic in Colicky Formula-Fed Infants: A Double-Blind Crossover Study," *Pediatrics* 1989; vol. 83, 2:262–266. The hazards of giving infants apple juice are documented in "Apple Juice: An Unappreciated Cause of Chronic Diarrhea," by Jeffrey S. Hyams and A. Leichtner, *American Journal of Diseases of Children* 1985; 139:503–5. Jeffrey S. Hyams, M.D., et al. documented children's difficulty absorbing sorbitol in *American Journal of Diseases of Children* 1985; 139:503. The Natural Resources Defense Council published its report on Alar in February 1989. Social custom as a factor in diet is discussed by Alan Silman and Jean Marr in their chapter, "A Better Western Diet: What Can Be Achieved?" in *Dietary Fibre, Fibre-Depleted Foods and Disease*, edited by Hugh C. Trowell, Denis Burkitt, and Kenneth Heaton (New York: Academic Press, 1985). Herbert M. Shelton's prescription of a daily salad appears in *Food Combining Made Easy* (San Antonio, Texas: Willow Publishing, 1982).

Exercise
The September 1988 issue of *Vegetarian Journal* (P.O. Box 1463, Baltimore, Maryland 21203, (301)752-VEGV) is devoted to "The Vegetarian Athlete."

People Over 65
A good overview of older people's nutritional problems is provided by Judith Swarth, M.S., R.D., in *Seniors and Nutrition*, a booklet in the Health Media of America Nutrition Series (Health Media of America, Inc., 11300 Sorrento Valley Road, Suite 250, San Diego, California 92121).

A C K N O W L E D G M E N T S

My special gratitude to the many talented and dedicated people who inspired and contributed to this book. Among them are several pioneers in the prevention of digestive disorders: James C. Breneman, M.D.; Denis P. Burkitt, M.D.; William Crook, M.D.; the late Carlton Fredericks, Ph.D.; V. Alun Jones, M.D.; C. Orian Truss, M.D. I owe particular thanks also to three mentors: Sidney Baker, M.D.; Jeffrey S. Bland, Ph.D.; and Jonathan V. Wright, M.D. Several generous colleagues kindly provided ideas and research material: Donald O. Castell, M.D.; James A. Duke, Ph.D.; Daniel J. Dunphy, P.A.C.; Steven L. Fahrion, Ph.D.; John Fudens, D.V.M.; Daniel Gagnon; Leo Galland, M.D.; Cedric Garland, M.D.; De Lamar Gibbons, M.D.; Gary Hitzig, M.D.; Russell M. Jaffe, M.D.; Mr. and Mrs. V. E. Irons; David Mastroianni, Ph.D.; Daniel Present, M.D.; Khem M. Shahani, Ph.D.; Gabriel Stux, M.D.; Gérard V. Sunnen, M.D.; and Dana Ullman, M.P.H. I especially appreciate the careful readings and critiques that Charles Stimler, M.D., and Kirk Zachary, M.D., gave my manuscript. My gratitude also goes to Steve and Sarah C. Bell; David Camhi, D.C.; Ria Eagan, D.C.; Sara C. Lee; Betty Morelli; Julie Motz; Cathy Sears; the staffs of the National Center for Health Statistics and the New York Academy of Medicine Library; and the staff and patients of the Hoffman Center for Holistic Medicine. Finally, I am deeply grateful for the unending patience, invaluable help, and unfailing support of my agent, Anne Borchardt, and my editor, Fred C. Hills. I owe special thanks to Ann Marie Cunningham, without whom this book would not exist, and to my wife, Helen Burgess, without whom I would not exist.

Index

colon cancer (*cont.*)
  fat intake and, 66, 237–38
  fiber and, 102, 237–38
  flora in, 41
  Hemoccult test and, 148–49
  iron and, 238
  macrobiotic diet and, 240–41
  surgery for, 138
  symptoms of, 237
  vegetables and, 238–39
  vitamin C and, 239–40
  yogurt and, 240
colonics, 195–97
colonoscopy, 148–49, 196, 197
colostomy, 138, 226
colostrum, 41, 216
comfrey tea, 140
comprehensive digestive stool
    analysis (CDSA), 147–48, 151
constipation, 15, 16, 45, 46, 75, 91,
    101, 102, 119, 134, 141, 144,
    192–97
  causes of, 72, 193–94
  colonics and, 195–97
  defined, 192
  gas and, 187
  herb tea and, 140
  laxatives and, 18, 193, 194–95,
    214, 215, 253–54
  in older people, 194
  in women, 193–94
  see also irritable bowel syndrome
cooking, food poisoning and, 245
coprolites, 143
cortisone, 92
cramping, 75
crash diets, 44, 234
Crile, George, 45, 211
Crohn's disease, 138, 146, 224–25,
    226
cruciferous vegetables, 117, 239
cytoprotection, 35–37, 44, 57, 60,
    217, 218
Cytotec, 219

dairy products, 59, 66, 75
  diarrhea and, 215
  food poisoning from, 243–44
  intolerance to, 75, 78–85; *see also*
    lactose intolerance

unpasteurized, traveler's diarrhea
    and, 247
decaffeinated coffee, 57
deglutition, 34
detoxification, 155
diaphragmatic breathing, 167–68
diarrhea, 41, 42, 44, 45, 46, 63, 75,
    91, 117, 120, 125, 133, 162,
    211–17
  acute, 211–12
  alcohol and, 60–61, 214
  chronic, as indication of serious
    illness, 211
  dehydration in, 46, 212
  determining cause of, 212–14
  fatty, 89, 138
  feces consistency and, 146
  gas and, 187
  in infants, 41, 46, 212, 214, 251
  during menstruation, 134, 135
  prophylactics against, 132
  running and, 167
  traveler's, 44, 46, 131–32, 213,
    246–48
  treatment of, 173, 214–17
  vitamin C and, 140
  see also irritable bowel syndrome
dietetic foods, 140, 214
dieting, 44, 61, 164, 234
Di-Gel, 186, 187
digestive tract, 28–42
  acidity in, 149–50
  defenses of, 29, 30, 34, 40
  diagram of, 33
  efficiency of, 30
  journey of food in, 31–42
  locations of organs in, 32
  perpetual motion in, 28–29; *see*
    also peristalsis
  traveling times in, 33; *see also*
    transit time
  see also specific organs
digestive troubles, 43–47
  body as source of clues about,
    141–43
  detective work on, 124–53
  fecal analysis and, 143–49
  risk factors for, 126–41
  tests for, 147–52
  see also specific problems

Imodium, 201, 215
indigestion, 15, 44, 75, 91, 162, 253
  alcohol and, 60
  see also heartburn
infant formulas, 250
infants, 29, 250–52
  breast-feeding of, 214, 250–51
  diarrhea in, 41, 46, 212, 214, 251
  gastrocolic reflex in, 47
infections:
  diarrhea and, 212
  ulcers and, 127, 220–21
  vaginal or urinary tract, 64, 91,
    136
  see also parasitic infections
inflammatory bowel disease (IBD),
    88, 224–30
  causes of, 226
  Crohn's disease and, 138, 146,
    224–25, 226
  dietary treatment of, 226–29
  mysteries about, 229–30
  surgical treatment of, 138, 225–26
  symptoms of, 224–25
  ulcerative colitis and, 46, 138, 146,
    224, 225–26
insulin, 135
intestinal bypass surgery, 44, 137,
    138–39
intestines, *see* colon; small intestine
intolerances, *see* food intolerances
involuntary (autonomic) nervous
    system, 42–43, 135, 164
iron, 253
  absorption of, 71, 136
  cancer and, 238
  megadoses of, 159
Irons, V. E., 196, 197, 199
irritable bowel syndrome (IBS), 45,
    47, 58, 75, 86, 102, 127, 135,
    140, 171, 200–208, 212, 213
  causes of, 200–201
  constipation in, 193, 194, 201
  diarrhea in, 201, 212, 214
  dietary changes and, 203–4
  exercise and, 167, 208
  feces consistency and, 146
  food intolerances and, 88, 89, 203–
    204
  gas and, 183

Giardia infections mistaken for,
    130, 133, 202
  herbal remedies for, 204–5
  in infants, 251
  medical treatment for, 201–3
  stress and, 162, 201, 205

Jaffe, Russell, 148
Japanese food:
  colon cancer and, 110–11
  miso, 123
  parasites in, 128–29, 244
  seaweed, 115–17
jejunum, *Giardia* in, 152
Jones, V. Alun, 203
junk food, 44, 68–70, 252

Kaopectate, 215
kidneys, 112
  antacids and, 71–72
kidney stones, 44, 72, 138, 141
Koch, Robert, 247
kombu, 186
Konsyl, 194
Koop, C. Everett, 51, 53
kudzu (kuzu), 119–20
Kushi, Michio, 160, 241
Kyolic, 118

Lactaid, 82–83
lactase, 126
lactobacilli, 85, 120, 122–23, 132,
    216–17, 240
Lactobacillus acidophilus, 85, 240
  see also acidophilus
lactose, 63
  foods containing, 81–82
lactose intolerance, 76, 78, 80–83,
    84–85, 99, 131, 212
  coping with, 82–83, 85
  gas and, 183–84
  incidence of, in adults, 80
  in infants, 251
  irritable bowel syndrome and, 203
large intestine, *see* colon
lassi, 122
laxatives, 18, 193, 194–95, 214, 215,
    253–54
leaky gut syndrome, 128
legumes, *see* beans

Quinacrine, 152
quinoa, 90

Rabelais, François, 254
rectal swab test, 151
red meat, food poisoning from, 244
refrigeration, 245
rejuvelac, 123
Relaxation Response, The (Benson),
163, 177
relaxation techniques, 163–70
    biofeedback, 164, 173–75
    breathing, 164, 167–68
    exercise, 164, 166–67
    meditation, 11, 161, 164, 169–70,
    205
    muscle, 164, 169–70
    self-hypnosis, 164, 175–77
    starting program of, 165–66
restaurants, food poisoning in, 244–
    245
rhubarb, 20, 112, 194–95
"runner's reflux," 167, 191, 208, 252

saccharin, 63
St. Martin, Alexis, 29–30, 42
saliva, 30, 32, 34, 36, 39, 41, 44, 60,
    118, 161
Salmonella, 128, 134, 136, 139, 243–
    244, 245, 246
salt, 25, 117
saturated fats, 66, 67
sauerkraut, 123
Schwartz, Mark, 165
seaweed, 115–17
seeds, 87, 186
self-hypnosis, 164, 175–77
serotonin, 59
sex factor, digestive troubles and,
    134–36
Shahani, Khem, 85, 216, 240
Shaw, George Bernard, 160
Shaw, Henry Wheeler, 154
shellfish, food poisoning from, 244
Shelton, Herbert M., 156–57, 158,
    252
shopping, food poisoning and, 245
short-gut syndrome, 138
Shurtleff, William, 119–20, 123
simethicone, 186, 187

Sinequan, 202
small intestine, 32, 33, 36, 38–40
    alcohol and, 59, 60
    celiac sprue and, 88–90, 125, 146
    coffee and, 57
    immune system of, 44–45
    nutrient absorption in, 38, 39, 44,
    59
    surface of, 38–39
small-intestine bypass, 44, 137, 138–
    139
smoking, 51–54
    cancer and, 51–52, 53
    colitis and, 229
    esophageal trouble and, 53
    heartburn and, 52, 53, 191
    stopping of, 53–54
    stress and, 164
    ulcers and, 52, 219
sodium bicarbonate, 72
sorbitol, 63, 140, 184, 214
spastic colon, *see* irritable bowel
    syndrome
spices, ulcers and, 221–22
sprouting beans and seeds, 186
starch blockers, 122, 155
steroids, 64, 225
stomach, 31, 32, 33, 35–37, 39, 43,
    53, 59, 118
    acid secreted by, 35, 37, 38, 41,
    43–44, 52, 57, 60, 71, 113–14,
    125–26, 136, 142, 149–50, 253
    coffee and, 57
    self-protective mechanism of, 35–
    37, 44, 57, 60, 217, 218
    surgery on, 137–38
    see also ulcers
stomach cancer, 53, 239, 240
    allium vegetables and, 117–18
stool, *see* bowel movements; feces
Stout, Rex, 74, 100
stress, 43, 45, 57, 73, 127, 140, 161–
    177
    charting in food diary, 165
    homeopathy and, 171–73
    inflammatory bowel disease and,
    230
    irritable bowel syndrome and, 162,
    201, 205
    physiological effects of, 162–63